THE
MAGICAL
AND
RITUAL
USE
OF
APHRODISIACS

D0770127

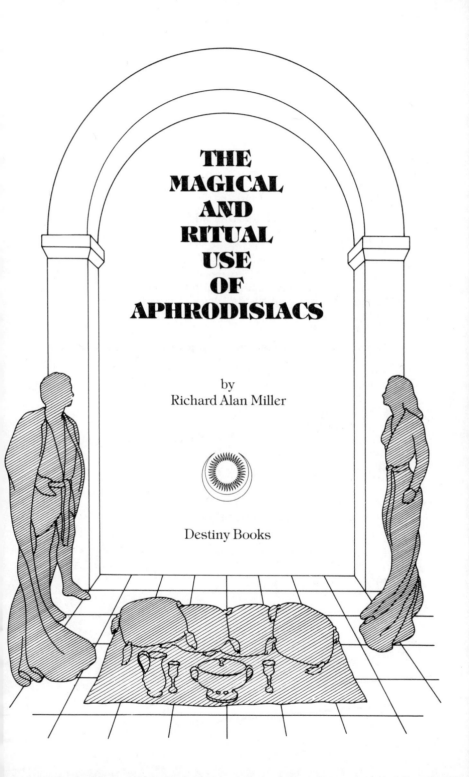

THE MAGICAL AND RITUAL USE OF APHRODISIACS

by
Richard Alan Miller

Destiny Books

Destiny Books
377 Park Avenue South
New York, New York 10016

Copyright © 1985 Richard Alan Miller

Text illustrations by Connie Nygard

Library of Congress Cataloging in Publication Data

Miller, Richard Alan, 1944
   The magical and ritual use of aphrodisiacs.

   Bibliography: p.
   Includes index.
   1. Aphrodisiacs. 2. Psychotropic plants. 3. Psycho-
tropic plants—Folklore. I. Title.
HQ12.M55   1985   615'.766   84-17003
ISBN 0-89281-062-9 (pbk.)

Destiny Books is a division of
Inner Traditions International Ltd.

Printed and bound in Great Britain

10 9 8 7 6 5 4 3 2 1

Dedication

To my wife, Iona

"I shall show you a love philtre without medicaments, without herbs, without a witche's incantations. It is this: If you want to be loved, then you must love first."

— Medieval folklore

Contents

PART II

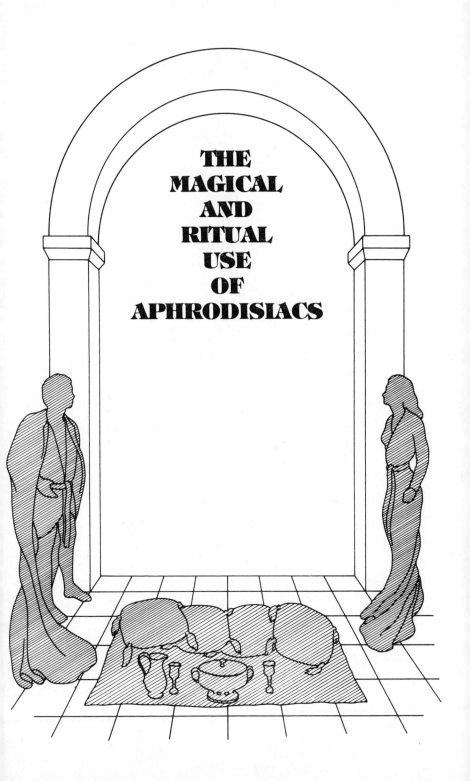

THE MAGICAL AND RITUAL USE OF APHRODISIACS

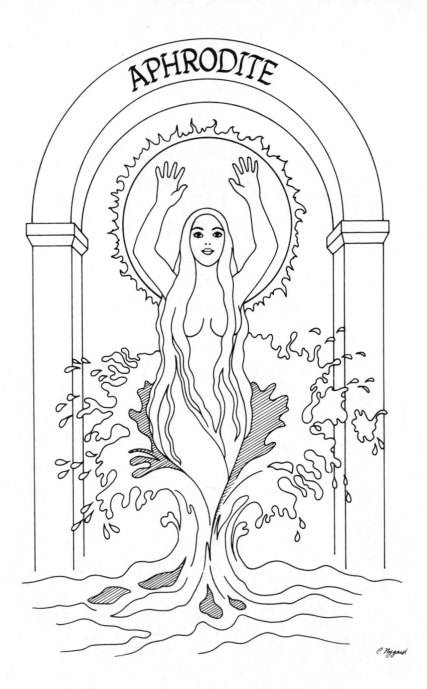

Introduction

The quest for a true aphrodisiac—some potion, pill, or food that guarantees better sex or bigger orgasms — is as old as man, woman, or even sex itself. Throughout history man has tried various means in which to enhance sexuality, although it is questionable as to whether these means delivered what they promised.

Some of the earliest known edible aphrodisiacs were popular because it was assumed that eating things that resembled our sexual organs would boost our sexual performance. This was known as the "doctrine of signatures," from Culpepper's book of the sixteenth century, and included such foods as clams, oysters, eggs, asparagus, bananas, and rhinoceros horn.

Because much of our sexuality is psychological in nature, man did not necessarily feel cheated, since even the suggestion of taking an "aphrodisiac" may create a placebo effect. However, since man is today seen as a biochemical creature, there is a need to contemporize our understanding of what the word aphrodisiac implies. It is interesting to note that even with the increased availability of sex in our times, the search for the one perfect sex stimulant has not diminished.

The word aphrodisiac comes from the name of Aphrodite, the Greek goddess of love and beauty. She is not only a goddess of fertility in the usual sense, but is also one of fertile imagination. By way of definition, an aphrodisiac should do one of the following:

1. Produce erections in the male,
2. Arouse sexual feelings by stimulation of the genitals or nervous system,
3. Increase sexual awareness,
4. Relax inhibitions,
5. Augment physical energy,
6. Strengthen the gonads or other glands involved with sex,
7. Improve sexual health,
8. Increase the production of semen,
9. Help conquer impotence and frigidity,
10. Overcome sexual exhaustion, or
11. Prevent premature ejaculation.

Those "love foods" that do work fall mainly into two classifications, biochemical aphrodisiacs which have a direct effect on sexual activity, and the more important psychophysical group. The psychophysical group of foods are by no means less effective but owe their potency partly to man's ancient belief in the therapeutic efficacy of resemblance. According to this notion, the gods left a mark on every plant to show the use for which it had been created.

There is no sexual organ more important than the human mind. There is no physical and mental experience or sensation complex more ecstatic and blissful than an ideal and complete sexual union between two loving partners. There are no anaphrodisiacs, dampeners, or desexualizers worse than ignorance, anxiety, or fear regarding the quality and effectiveness of one's performance of the sex act. The greatest sexual tonic is experienced when the physical and psychic personalities are in balance and the body can spontaneously respond from a depth of feeling.

People generally attribute to sex the two functions of procreation and recreation. But sex offers much more than the limited ecstasy of orgasm or the satisfaction of perpetuation of the species. Orgasm can easily be achieved through masturbation and procreation by means of artificial insemination. Sex is not mere lust, even if lust is sex. It transcends the two major animal functions and enters the realm of the cultural and spiritual. When combined with ritual, sex can accelerate progress toward cultural refinement and spiritual health.

Every act that soothes and satisfies an individual without resulting in an adverse reaction later on, and which promotes feelings of love, consideration, solicitude, constitutes progress toward culture and spirituality. Therefore, a proper exercise of a healthy sex urge, viewed from a detached, scientific perspective, is not only compatible with higher social, cultural, and spiritual goals but is actually conducive to them.

Nature has endowed women with a very convenient apparatus for practicing deception in sexual intercourse. In this matter men have been sadly let down by nature. If a man hates a woman, in most cases he will not be able to have an erection, the essential prerequisite to full intercourse. A greater tragedy for a man occurs when he is genuinely attracted to a woman but is unable to have an erection because of fear and anxiety.

The main disorders that plague men—lack of erection, premature ejaculation, absence of seminal discharge at the time of orgasm, or the absence of the orgasm itself—are, in most cases, psychological in origin, just as are frigidity and fear of coitus in women. Regular practice of ritual helps to tone up not only the neuromuscular structure of the organs concerned, but also helps steady and rehabilitate the mind.

When the demands of sex on the physical faculties become excessive in frequency and intensity, replenishment of energy is necessary. These are cases in which "the spirit is willing, but the flesh is weak." Substances that arouse and intensify the sex urge, even when one has low energy, are called aphrodisiacs. A woman takes about four times as long as a man to become fully

5

stimulated for the enjoyment of sex. The ritual use of aphrodisiacs controls haste in a man and gives him time to wait with patience until the urge of the female joins his. This results in greater benefit and pleasure for both.

A thorough knowledge of the chemical properties and specific effects of various aphrodisiacs prevents disappointment and the wasting of money and energy. During the past few years, several companies have offered aphrodisiacs for sale at outrageous prices with "guaranteed" results. Some of these promises are rather overstated in view of the following facts.

1. Impotence, frigidity, and premature ejaculation are usually of pathological origin.

2. When physical debility interferes with erection, potency, staying power, or enjoyment, the problem is usually best overcome by correction in nutrition, adequate rest, reduction of tension, or suitable exercise.

3. Although some of the materials discussed in this book, such as ginseng and gotu kola, are beneficial to health and can be taken regularly, many others are powerful drugs that may be valuable on occasion but should not be continued to a point of dependency.

The purpose of this book is to identify what these aphrodisiac substances are, where they can be found and what they look like, what their particular history is, and to give a complete chemical description and preparation and then offer a contemporary ritual designed to use them in an even more correct fashion for a contemporary application of their chemistry. It is my hope that the reader will learn from this text how to best use — not abuse — the aphrodisiacs described.

I am not prescribing any of these substances, legal or otherwise, for the reader. I can therefore not be held responsible for any mishap or failure that may occur through the use or misuse of any of these materials or the information that has been supplied.

PART I

"Medea gather'd the enchanted herbs
That did renew old Aeson."
Shakespeare, *The Merchant of Venice*

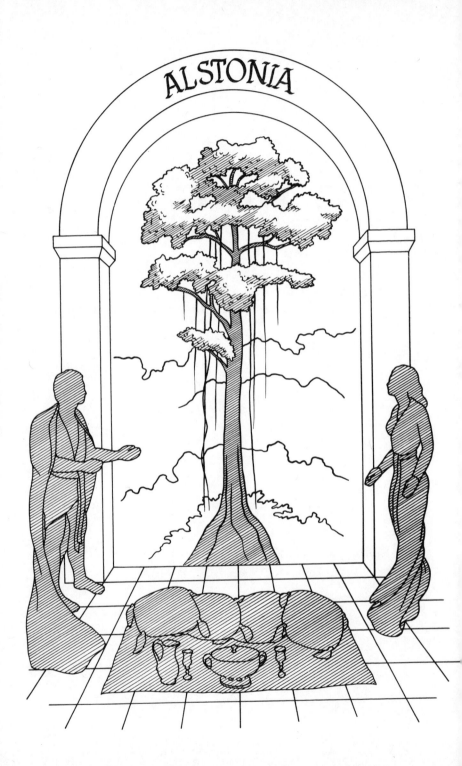

*Helps retain erection and delays orgasm
during intercourse*

Alstonia

Family: Apocynaceae.

Botanical Name: *Alstonia scholaris.*

Synonyms: Dita, bitter bark, devil's tree, pale mara, chhatim (India).

Geographical Location: Eastern Asia, India, and the Philippines.

Habitat: Tropical rain forests of India, Ceylon, and Borneo.

Botanical Description: The Dita tree grows from 50 to 80 feet in height and has a furrowed trunk. Being part of the dogbane family, it has oblong, stalked leaves up to 6 inches long and 4 inches wide. The upper side of the leaf is glossy and the under side is white, with nerves running at right angles to the mid-rib. The bark is odorless and very bitter to the taste, and is brownish-grey with blackish spots on the outer side. The Dita tree has white, funnel-shaped flowers.

History: The bark rolls off the tree in layers that have long been used by Asian scholars as a kind of parchment on which to write. It was this usage that led to its Latin last name, *scholaris*. The bark has also been used in Asian folk medicine for ages. A tea made from the bark has long been a standard and effective method for lessening the distress of menstrual cramps. In current homeopathic practice a tea made of the bark and seeds is used to cure chronic diarrhea and dysentery. The bark, however, has no aphrodisiacal properties.

Chemistry: The bark contains three alkaloids, ditamine, echitamine (ditaine), and echitenines. There are also several fatty and resinous substances; both bases resemble ammonia in chemical characteristics. The seed contains a powerful alkaloid, chlorogenine $(C_{21}H_{20}N_2O_4)$, now considered the principle agent that acts as an aphrodisiac. Chlorogenic acid may not be the aphrodisiac first believed but may act more as a universal allergen. It is widespread in many plants and is concentrated in coffee beans and castor beans.

Reserpine has also been reported in *Alstonia constricta,* a variation of the Dita tree. Reserpine and other *Rauvolfia* alkaloids act on the sympathetic nervous system by depleting most of the neurotransmitter substance norepinephrine. This neural locking results in an overabundance of serotonin (see Hormones, pages 123-132).

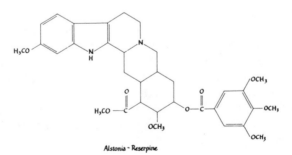

Alstonia - Reserpine

Primary Effects: The chlorogenic acid causes minor irritation of the genitals, stirring up erotic energies in the form of tingling sensations in the genito-urinary tract. It will also prolong erection and delay orgasm, acting as a general tonic and mild stimulant for the nerves and circulation.

Preparation: Begin with crushing two grams of seeds and soaking them in two ounces of water overnight. The following day the liquid is strained and drunk. The exact dosages must be determined on the basis of both the alkaloid potency in a particular batch of seeds and the individual's drug tolerance. Increase the dosage a little at a time as needed.

Ritual Use: It was in *tantric* India that the seed of the dita tree was first used as an aphrodisiac. Use of the drug was accompanied by an exercise that prolonged erection and delayed orgasm by control of specific genital muscles.

The exercise is excellent for improving the elasticity of the genital muscles and at the same time puts them under voluntary control. You can do this exercise in any position, anywhere. It is an excellent exercise because it not only massages the prostate gland in males, but also increases control of the genital muscles in females. This ancient tantric exercise strengthens the puboccygeus muscle, which passes from the pubic bone at the front of the pelvis box to the coccyx, or tailbone, in the back.

This muscle operates in the same way as a circular valve and is the same muscle that opens and closes the three apertures in the lower torso. These apertures cannot be controlled separately in independent muscles, but one can exercise to the degree that one can focus the main effort on only one of the openings. In this way one can gain voluntary control and make it more flexible by the following daily exercises.

11

1. Relax as if urinating, but then firmly contract the muscles as if to stop the flow.

2. Release the urine as usual, then contract the muscle to stop the flow.

3. Observe the muscle used.

4. Hold the muscle in contraction for a second or two, and then release.

5. Do it again.

In many cultures this exercise is used by the female partner to stimulate vaginal orgasm and to heighten sexual pleasure for her partner.

Note of caution: *Chlorogenic acid is a universal allergen and acts as an irritant to the bladder and genitals.*

In Ceylon its light wood is used for coffins.

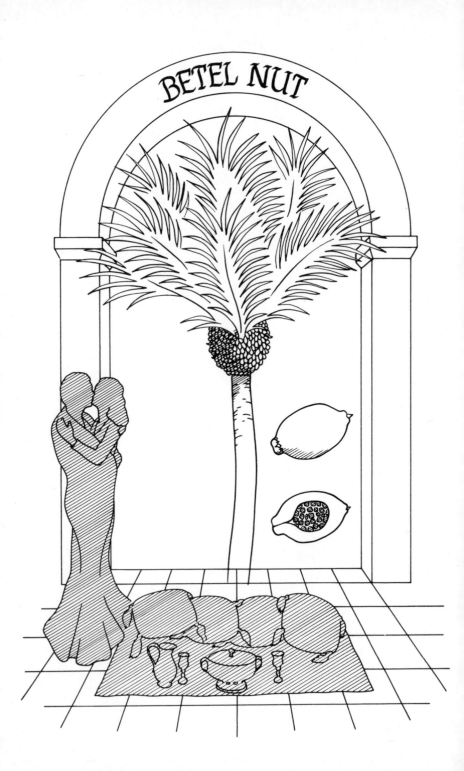

Betel Nut

Family: Palmaceae (Palm).

Botanical Name: *Areca catechu.*

Synonyms: areca nut, pinang, siri, suprari (Hindu), ping lang (Chinese).

Geographical Location: India, Malay, and Polynesia.

Habitat: Grows everywhere in the South Pacific islands.

Botanical Description: A slender climbing tree that grows to 75 feet in height. The trunk is ringed and is usually trained on poles or trellises in hot, shady environments. The leaves grow to be as much as three feet across, with many pinnae (it is a compound leaf with many divisions separated by veins).

History: By the 1930's it was estimated that at least 20,000,000 persons chewed betel nuts in India alone. Each betel palm produces about 250 seeds or nuts per year, and millions of these trees are under cultivation. It is one of the world's most popular plants, with the leaf used as a paper for rolling tobacco. The regular use of betel nuts does, in time, stain the mouth, gums, and teeth a deep red. Asian betel chewers, however, are quite proud of these stains.

The Malayan technique for using betel nut is to mix a mashed or powdered nut, some catechu gum from the Malayan acacia tree (*Acacia catechu*), a pinch of burnt lime, and a dash of nutmeg, cardamom, or turmeric for flavor. This mash is then rolled up in a leaf from the betel vine (*Piper chavica betel*). These rolls are sold on the streets or in markets as candy.

Chemistry: Arecoline, a volatile oil, is released from the nut by saliva and lime (calcium oxide). Betel leaf contains chavicol, allylpyrocathechol, chavibetol, and cadinese. Arecoline is in the same cholinergic alkaloid group as is muscarine, found in *Amanita muscaria* (Fly Agaric).

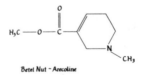

Betel Nut – Arecoline

Primary Effects: Arecoline is a mild central nervous system (CNS) stimulant. It increases respiration while decreasing the work load on the heart.

Preparation: Mix 1/2 gram of burnt lime (hydrated calcium oxide) with one betel nut, preferably in a semi-powdered form. Place in the side of the mouth, like a plug of tobacco, for a two-hour period. Spit the saliva occasionally.

16

Ritual Use: The CNS stimulant effects seem to make time pass more quickly. The herb is perfect for times of posture meditation or when learning control of the body. The ability to control the body is important (as is controlling thoughts) when performing tantric sex magic rituals. This form of control is known as asana, or posture.

With a mild stimulant, difficult postures may be maintained longer, and the time seems to "fly by" rather than drag. The following exercises are used in the development of control in posture. When doing the exercises, wear no constricting garments. Learn to sit perfectly still with every muscle tense for long periods of time.

1. The first position (The God): Sit in a chair with head up, back straight, knees together, hands on knees, and eyes closed.
2. The second position (The Dragon): Kneel and rest the buttocks on the heels, toes turned back, back and head straight, and hands on thighs.
3. The third position (The Ibis): Stand, holding the left ankle with the right hand, and with the free forefinger on your lips.
4. The fourth position (The Thunderbolt): Sit with the left heel pressing up the anus; the right foot is poised on its toes, the heel covering the phallus; the arms are stretched out over the knees; the head and back are straight.

Various things will begin to happen to you while practicing these positions. They should be carefully analysed and described in a journal. Note the duration of each practice. The severity of the pain (if any) and the degree of rigidity attained should also be recorded, along with any other pertinent sensations.

When you have progressed to a point at which you feel confident with these exercises, place a saucer filled with water upon the head. You should eventually be able to poise this saucer on the head (while in a sitting posture) for at least one hour while doing these exercises.

Note of Caution: Excessive amounts of arecoline, from either overuse or the chewing of unripe areca nuts (which contain larger quantities of the oil), can cause inebriation, dizziness, and diarrhea. Prolonged usage can also cause damage to the teeth and soft tissue of the mouth.

Betel nut is considered an aphrodisiac because it stimulates one's available energy and elevates moods rather than directly influencing sexual organs. It is currently used like coffee (brewed) or cigarettes (smoked) in the United States and Europe.

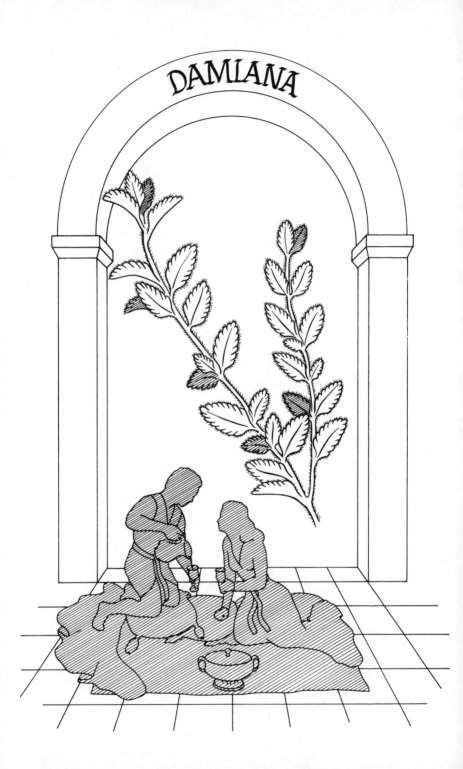

Damiana

Family: Turneraceae

Botanical Name: *Turnera diffusa* L.

Synonyms: Mexican damiana.

Geographical Location: Tropical parts of North America, particularly Texas and Mexico. It has also been harvested in Africa.

Habitat: Most deserts with dry soils and full sun.

Botanical Description: A small shrub with ovate leaves that broaden toward the top end. The leaves are smooth and pale green on the upper sides and smooth on the under sides except for a few hairs on the ribs. The flowers are yellow, arising singly from axila of the leaves, followed by a one-celled capsule splitting into three pieces. The flower has an aromatic smell with a bitter taste.

History: Damiana has been used for centuries by Mexican women. They found that a cup of damiana tea taken one or two hours before intercourse helped to immerse them in the sexual act. It was believed to have a tonic effect upon the sexual organs and the nervous system.

In his book, *A Manual of Sex Magick*, Louis J. Culling describes a drink that acts like a psychic aphrodisiac, made from dried damiana leaves and boiling water. Significant results would follow if used for several consecutive weeks. My companion book, *The Magical and Ritual Use of Herbs*, gives an excellent recipe for making an aphrodisiacal cordial of damiana and vodka. Both were used in Western forms of tantra, or sex magic.

Chemistry: Damiana leaves contain 0.2 to 0.9 percent volatile oil, 14 percent resin, approximately 3.5 percent tannin, 6 percent starch, and a bitter substance called damianian.

Primary Effects: The volatile oil is mildly irritating and may induce peristalsis and gentle stimulation of the genito-urinary tract during its excretion. Because of irritant action on the genito-urinary tract, it can be used to help rid the body of pre-existing urinary tract diseases. It is this mild irritation, causing stimulation, which makes it also act as a mild aphrodisiac. It also affects the psyche, producing a marijuana-like euphoria that can last for up to one and a half hours.

Preparation: To make a tea, take 2 heaping tablespoons of dried damiana leaf and place it in boiling water (1 cup) for less than 5 minutes. As a liqueur, the combination of damiana and vodka (1 ounce leaf to 1 pint of vodka for 5 days) makes an excellent psychic aphrodisiac that relaxes inhibitions. It has a bitter but aromatic taste and has been used as a mild purgative for years.

The following blend, known as Yuba Gold, should be used in a waterpipe and produces a "marijuana-like" high.

4 parts damiana leaf
4 parts scullcap herb
1/4 part lobelia herb
4 parts passion flower herb
1 part spearmint leaf

Ritual Use: Western forms of tantra include a series of sex magic rituals designed to bring the individual to self realization. The central aim of Western magic is to attain the "knowledge and conversation of the holy guardian angel," or the daemon, one's true spiritual identity. This implies drawing closer to the consciousness of one's real individuality, in contradistinction to the active conscious personality.

It thus becomes the aim of the aspirant in Western forms of tantra to be and to express one's true individuality as much as possible, instead of being submerged in the personality. Thus, the first practice undertaken by the neophyte (or beginner) is the development of contact with the subconscious mind.

By focusing on recalling our dreams we learn about our inner selves and can develop a clearer picture of our individual identities. We come to know ourselves, in the spiritual sense, as people composed of conflicting conscious and subconscious desires. Awareness of both leads to greater personal freedom and harmony through the synthesizing of aims.

One does not make any attempt to interpret the meaning of the dreams at the time of recording them. Over a two-month period, however, a code or cipher of symbols often emerges, shedding light on inner processes. Personal significance emerges by giving attention to the inner processes. Dreams reflect inner psychological changes. By giving them attention and recalling or recording them, conscious and subconscious begin to merge into a "borderland consciousness" that reflects individual wholeness. This is known as the magical identity.

The conscious ego learns to cooperate with the imaginative subconscious. The importance of the ability to function in a quasi-borderland state (neither awake nor profoundly asleep) may well be more than half of the technique of magic. It is involved in making the imagination seem subjectively real.

Alphaism is the first degree of sex magic. It is the practice of magical chastity wherein the magician has no emotions about sex between the occasions of sexual congress. One does not even fantasize actively about sex. It is not merely physical chastity that is of value. Rather, one reserves sexual interest and imagination for the time of actual sexual congress and its preparation. Sex magic places the sexual act upon a high, idealistic plane. It lifts sex play from the lowest plane of desire to the high plane of self-transformation.

The second degree of sex magic is called *Dianism*. Dianism is sexual congress without climax. The name is derived from that of the chaste goddess, Diana. The participants should be warm and ardent yet not allow themselves to be carried to the point of concupiscence. Practice in this art eventually produces a condition in which there is no sense of frustration even though orgasm is ruled out.

Rather than allowing oneself to be submerged in the full flow of pleasurable sensation, one should allow the ecstasy to feed the fires of aspiration and inspiration. The aim of *Dianism* and its highest magic lies in continuing the union until such time as one goes into the "borderland state," an imaginative realm neither fully conscious nor beyond control by the will. A damiana liqueur at this stage is perfect as a psychic aphrodisiac, rekindling the "flame" to prolong the borderland mood.

Here are some guidelines for this second degree of sex magic.

1. The required attitude of the partner aspiring to true individuality is to lose all possible awareness of the partner as a certain person. One should be as imper-

24

sonal as possible toward that personality.

2. The aspirant should regard the partner (imagined and visualized) as a tangible manifestation of his own daemon, his divine lover, transmuting the partner in imagination into a symbolic representative of divine inner forces.

3. The partner may have a climax only if it does not diminish continuing enjoyment of the borderland state. The partners should be relaxed, not sexually aggressive, and should never strive for the climax in a hurry.

4. They should welcome the ecstasy but should not indulge in it. Rather, they should imagine and will that the sexual ecstasy is immediately transformed into the continuing fire which feeds the magical visualization and imagination of being in union with one's soul lover. When this is done well, the desire for climax is repressed. Tantric yoga practice refrains from orgasm altogether, turning this energy toward psychological and spiritual creativity. One may not wish to practice this forever but might want to experiment with it during a time of needed change.

5. To create what is variously called the magical child, or the bud-will, continued acts of sex magic ritual are necessary. The processes of creativity and physical generation are analogous. Both require attraction, union, fertilization, incubation (or gestation), and birth. One's true or higher self must be formed by the union of conscious and subconscious energies that are nurtured and brought to birth after a period of containment. When the child is "born," the length of its life depends upon the force of the magical operation, symbolically expressing the strength of the psychological transformation process. This ritual should be performed every seven to nine days, increasing in strength to a maximum after three rites.

Note of Caution: *Excessive long-term use may be toxic to the liver.*

It was believed to be most effective when used in combination with saw palmetto berries (Serona repens) in a one to one ratio by weight.

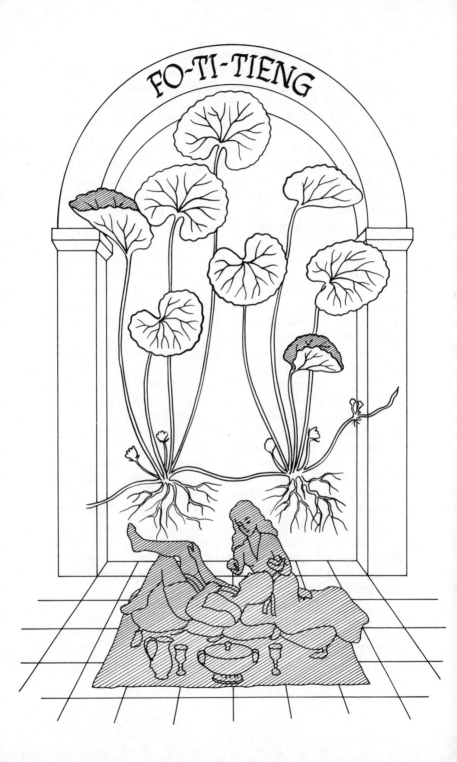

Fo-Ti-Tieng

Family: Umbelliferae (Parsley).

Botanical Name: *Hydrocotyle asiatica minor* L.

Synonyms: Asian march pennywort, Indian pennywort, boilean, bevilacqua, gotu kola.

Geographical Location: Throughout Asia and most of China. *Centella asiatica* (gotu kola) is a slightly larger geographical variant found in Ceylon, India, and parts of Africa. Often confused, they are *not* the same herb.

Habitat: Found growing wild along roadsides, on shady and damp hillsides, or in grass thickets.

Botanical Description: Perennial herb with a slender and delicate stem that creeps. Three to four leaves grow from nodes. They are ovate-rounded with rounded obtuse apexes. In summer, small, purple axillary flowers appear to form umbellate inflorescences. The fruit is flat-rounded and purplish red.

History: The fresh leaves of *Hydrocotyle asiatica minor* are eaten daily by many in Ceylon, primarily to

27

improve health and extend life. The plant was first noticed in the western world when several herb books cited the story of Li Chung Yun, a famous Chinese herbalist who died in 1933. He was reportedly born in 1677 and died at the age of 256. He was apparently living with his twenty-fourth wife at the time of his death.

One tends to doubt the accuracy of his birth and death records, but it is certain that the man did live an unusually long life, retaining his vigor to the very end. His diet included a strict vegetarian program and daily dosages of *fo-ti-tieng* and ginseng. Today a number of the sex-drug merchants promote the dried leaves of this Asian marsh pennywort as the very thing that bestowed this fabled longevity and sexual prowess upon Dr. Li Chung Yun.

The well-know French biochemist, Jules Lepine, found that the leaves and seeds from this plant contain an alkaloid with rejuvenating effects on the nerves, brain cells, and endocrine glands. Professor Menier of the Academie Scientifique near Paris made similar observations. It was noted that this substance stimulates a portion of the adrenal glands, which detoxify impurities in the body.

There is some contention among experts as to what Li's *fo-ti-tieng* actually was. The Chinese translates as "elixir of long life" and has been used freely on a number of other herbs, including gotu kola and fleece-flower root, as well as several concoctions of various herbs. Gotu kola is now considered a larger geographical variant of fo-ti-tieng and is sometimes called *Hydrocotyle asiatica major*.

Hydrocotyle is an Asian species of pennywort which is a low-growing type of herb. *Tieng* in Chinese means root, however. There is now some evidence to support the belief that the tuber (or root) of *Polygonium multiflori,* also known as Shoo Koo in Chinese, is fo-ti-tieng. The common name is fleeceflower root, and Dr. Leung Kok Yuen of the North American School of Acupuncture considers it to be the legendary fo-ti-tieng.

It has a history of many thousands of years of use in China.

Chemistry: The alkaloid extracted from the leaves and seeds of *Hydrocotyle asiatica minor* was called Vitamin X. Not much is known about this compound, although *Centella asiatica* is now used as an antibiotic. The extraction from gotu kola is asiaticoside, known to be an active agent against *tubercle bacilli.* Vitamin X is still relatively unknown.

Primary Effects: Daily use of 1/2 teaspoon of the powdered herb in a cup of hot water has excellent effects. These include improved digestion, resistance to certain diseases, calming of the nerves, increase in both physical and mental energies, and softening of signs of aging (like lines and wrinkles).

Larger amounts, such as 1 to 2 tablespoons daily, act as a sexual stimulant when the sexual vitality is low. Continued use has a beneficial cumulative effect on overall health.

Preparation: I recommend that fo-ti-tieng be taken daily. One technique is to cook 4 ounces of the leaf slowly (not boiling) for 6 hours and drink over 3 to 4 days, keeping 2 quarts of liquid in the cooking vessel.

Many people feel that the best results are experienced when fresh gotu kola leaves are used. The plant requires moderate shade and plenty of water. A few of the plants will send out runners and will spread like strawberries if conditions are just right. The leaves have a tangy flavor, and two or more should be chewed daily for the maintenance of vigor and as a psychic energizer.

Ritual Use: The Taoist secret of immortality could be summed up with the aphorism, "Master, do you ever emit?" "Only to make children." Even though Taoist magicians chose to foresake orgasms for immortality, they were left with a paradoxical dependence upon women for their process of transformation. Since they believed that the secretions of a woman's body contained the ingredients necessary to assure their immortality, these men were left with attitudes that simultaneously venerated and exploited women.

Ancient China was a patriarchal society which, nevertheless, believed that women were closer than men to immortal nature's primordial forces. Taoist magicians therefore alleged that sexual contact with as many women as possible (virgins were most preferred) would provide the sage with increased physical vigor, mental health, and longevity.

The transformation to an immortal state was thought accomplished through the blending of the yang element (semen) and the yin element (female secretions). The magician combined them in his own body, creating an infusion known as the nectar of immortality. An adept magician could induce his partner to several orgasms, thereby deriving maximal yin energy for his own transformation process. In order to accomplish his admittedly selfish goal, however, the man had to repress his own desire for orgasm and adhere perfectly to the rhythms of his current partner.

"Control a woman as you would a horse on a rotten rope." This quote from a Taoist sage sums up the sensitivity required for performing this type of magic successfully. But its benefits were not confined solely to male participants. A woman could also achieve immortality through this art form. The yin essence could be fulfilled by harmonizing with the yang. Women could gain transformative power by climaxing only rarely while exciting each of their partners to orgasm as many times as possible.

A woman having intercourse should quiet her mind and calm her heart. She should control her feelings in order to harmonize with her partner. She must not move wildly, thus causing herself to experience premature orgasm. If her yin energies are exhausted first, her body is considered empty and she may become susceptible to colds.

Taoist literature states that only very advanced yogic practitioners ought to refrain from orgasm altogether. In applying Taoist concepts to a contemporary life-style, we should be content to harmonize sincerely with our partner's motions and emotions, thereby creating our own prescription for a nectar of immortality, for the relationship, at least. One way to accomplish this is not to waste breath and keep all of the attention in the here and now of the experience.

Taoist sexual practice reaches its highest expression when both partners cooperate in a process of mutual transformation and melding of yin and yang energies. A famous Chinese legend recounts the benefits of a balanced exchange of sexual energies. Madam "Fairy" Koo was a woman of the Tang Dynasty (618-906) who gave as well as she received. She had three secret techniques which enhanced her art:

1. "Lowering the Recreation Chamber to greet the advancing Ambassador." This indicates that the woman sits astride the man and moves her hips in a circular, grinding motion. According to this legendary technique, she should then raise her body and pause momentarily, gripping the male organ so that it hangs beneath her "like an animal in the claws of an eagle."

2. "Raising the Recreation Chamber to climb up to the Ambassador." The woman reclines on her back and adheres perfectly to the man's rhythmical movements. Either she can meet his forward thrusts with equally strong ones of her own, creating deep soft collisions, or she may coordinate her undulations with her partner's, thus eliminating all sensations of friction. The latter skill is specifically used to prolong the man's pleasure and create an "oceanic" experience in the psyche of both participants.

3. "Bursting of the Clouds," or orgasm. For this, the woman should position herself so that the semen flows directly into the uterus, seizing the "turtle's head" with her interior muscles by contracting the sphincter muscle of the vagina. At this point, she should urge her

31

partner to remain still so that both experience the subtle aspects of the moment. The yang essence flowing from his penis and the yin essence from her excretions can flow simultaneously past each other in a perfect exchange of vital sexual fluids. This amalgam, known as the nectar of immortality, is then imagined as raised up the spine into the cranium where it exerts a psychological transformation on the consciousness.

As you coordinate with your partner's movements and breath, your combined circulation of energy is increased, and more power is accumulated for the eventual orgasm. *Consciousness is the key factor.* You must keep your whole mind in the here and now throughout the act, not fantasizing, not striving, just feeling, and holding back from orgasm without dropping your concentration. When the "bursting of the clouds" finally overwhelms you, it can be a truly transforming experience. This is the magic of the alchemy of the Taoist.

Note of Caution: *There seems to be a great difference of opinion regarding what is the true fo-ti-tieng, of Dr. Li. None of the discussed possible herbs have any reported toxicities; all have some traditional use as elixers of long life.*

The original folk use of gotu kola *(Centella asiatica)* was as a treatment for leprosy. There now seems to be some correlation with that disease and the antibiotic action of this plant. Gotu kola has also been used to prevent nervous breakdowns. And as a youth-prolonging drug the Sinhalese have a saying about the herb: "Two leaves a day keep old age away."

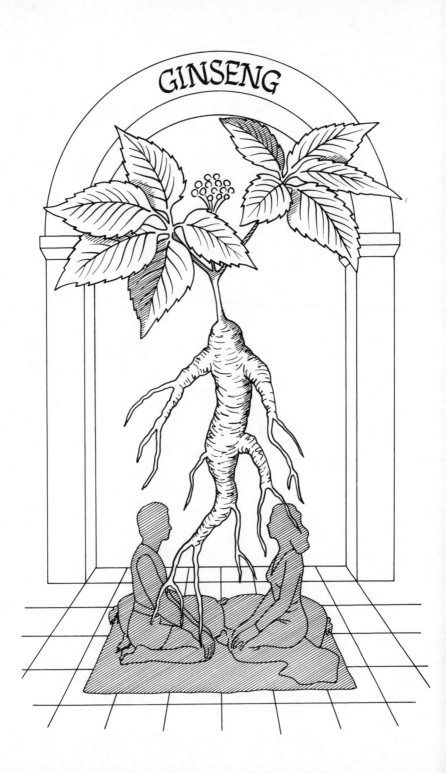

Ginseng

Family: Araliaceae.

Botanical Name: *Panax quinquefolium L.*

Synonyms: American ginseng, sang, redberry, five-fingers, divine root, root of life, man root.

Geographical Location: Found in the wild from Maine to Minnesota and south to the mountains of northern Georgia and Arkansas. Ginseng has also long been cultivated in small areas in the northern and central States and in the Pacific Northwest.

Habitat: It is found sparingly in the rich, moist soils of hardwood forests.

Botanical Description: Ginseng is an erect plant growing from 8 to 15 inches in height and bearing three leaves at its summit. Each leaf consists of five thin, stalked leaflets. The three upper ones are larger than the two lower ones. Six to twenty greenish-yellow flowers are produced in a small cluster during July and August, followed later in the season by bright crimson berries.

Ginseng has a thick, fleshy, spindle-shaped root 2 to 3 inches or more in length and about one-half to 1 inch in diameter, often branched. After the second year the root becomes branched or forked, and it is the branched root, especially if it resembles the human form, which finds particular favor with the Chinese, the principal consumers of the root.

History: The Chinese have been fascinated by the "man plant" for over 5,000 years. Like mandrake, the most potent ginseng roots are said to be shaped like a man's body. The Chinese further believed that even better results were obtained when the root was dug up at midnight during a full moon. Oriental men have consumed this root daily for over 5,000 years in order to retain their virility. An ancient medical manuscript of India says of ginseng that it "bestows on men both young and old the power of a bull" (Atherva Veda).

Indian tribes of the United States first learned of the virtues of ginseng in the sixteenth century. Entire tribes would harvest the abundant *Panax quinquefolium,* the North American species of this root crop. The Meskwakis Indians, for example, were known to concoct a special love potion with these harvests, combining it with mica, snake meat, gelatin, and some wild columbine herb. A young girl of the tribe would use the mixture to find a husband by feeding it to an unsuspecting male.

A Chinese *materia medica* of the fourth century presented a list of exotic ginseng recipes which supposedly increased sexual appetites. Shen-Nung, one of the first Chinese emperors to practice alchemy and the use of sex for rejuvenation, recorded that he felt warmth and sexual desire after chewing some of the root. Ginseng's reputation as an aphrodisiac, however, owes most of its power to "The Doctrine of Signatures" (a philosophy based on form, color, and so on), since it has a phallic shape.

Chemistry: Six glycosides (acetal derivatives of sugar)

called panaxosides have been isolated from ginseng. Most significant are the four major sapogenins (those structures attached to the glycosides), which can be "cleved" from the root. They are panaquilon, panaxapogenol, panaxin, and panacene.

The stimulating effects of these sapogenins do not fully explain the potency of ginseng as a tonic or clinical drug. They merely facilitate the effects of the two remaining sapogenins, panaxadiol and panaxatriol. These are chemically triterpene constructed; they possess an isometric hydrocarbon structure ($C_{10}H_{16}$) prevalent in many medicinal plants. They are used especially as a solvent in organic synthesis. Panaxatriol is present in the root, while panaxadiol is present in the root extract.

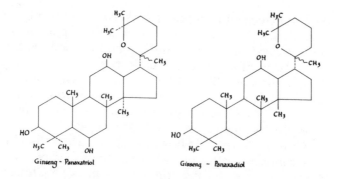

Ginseng - Panaxatriol   Ginseng - Panaxadiol

Ginseng is also rich in vitamins B_1 and B_2 and contains the minerals phosphorus, iron, aluminum, copper, manganese, cobalt, sulfur, and silica. These are present in the glutaninin acids and the amylase and phenolase enzymes. It is the steroid nucleus of ginseng, however, which is significantly different from most other plants. This may be the key to explaining ginseng's amazing regulatory and curative properties.

According to the *Cyclopedia Dictionary of Medical Botany of the USSR* by G. S. Ogolovec (1955), ginseng also gives off minute amounts of a unique type of ultraviolet radiation that stimulates the healthy growth of tissue, especially in the endocrine system. This subtle radioactive quality is known as "mitogenic radiation." Russian researchers make a fluid extract from Siberian ginseng *(Eleutherococcus senticosis),* which is widely distributed to the public. Russian astronauts took this drug, which is not a true ginseng, to strengthen them in their hazardous venture.

Primary Effects: Panaquilon stimulates and increases endocrine activity. Panaxapogenol (panax acid) promotes a mild increase in metabolic activity and relaxes heart and artery movements. Panaxin stimulates the central organs, heart, and blood vessels. Panacene stimulates the medulla centers and relaxes the central nervous system.

Preparation: Ginseng can be taken in a number of different ways. It is best taken by chewing a piece about the thickness of a pencil and 1 inch in length. Saliva helps activate its qualities; simply swallowing capsules is not as efficient. The Chinese make a tea by boiling 1 teaspoon of the root filaments in a pint of water for 10 minutes. The pulp is not wasted but is used several more times and is then chewed and swallowed.

Ginseng tea should be sipped slowly, thus allowing it to combine with the salivary fluids before swallowing. Another form is the very expensive Chinese wine called *kaoliang,* with ginseng roots soaked in its cask for at least three years. As strong as vodka, it is usually taken in a small glass as a nightcap.

An old French recipe for a love wine that can be made at home uses ginseng. In two pints of Chablis, crush an ounce of vanilla bean, one of cinnamon chips, one of dried rhubarb, and one of ginseng (or alternatively, mandrake). Leave to stand for two weeks and stir daily. It is then strained through cheesecloth and a small amount of amber is added for color.

Ritual Use: Daily intake of ginseng as a general sexual tonic might be considered by some as important a daily ritual as brushing one's teeth. It certainly formed an intrinsic part of the Taoist orientation toward sex. Even if we do not apply all of the Taoist axioms in our lovemaking practices these days, we can still benefit from using ginseng to add more zest to our lives.

Taoist magicians believed in the importance of balancing male (yang) and female (yin) elements in the act of love. They felt that if the lovers were in "harmony," it nourished both of the partners, bringing them closer to the spirit of the universe. When the partners were in balance, neither strove for pleasure *independently* of the other.

We can make use of the Taoist attitude in our encounters today by keeping this principle in mind. This does not mean making a fetish out of simultaneous orgasms. However, the Taoists contended that the "life force" was contained within the byproducts of the orgasm (i.e., semen and vaginal fluids). Therefore, in order to maintain balance, we require the complementary yin or yang energies of our partner. The Taoist system recommends that men and women yield these complementary energies to one another. Then yin and yang blend, nourishing both parties and increasing health and longevity.

For the Taoists, orgasm was only one aspect of the interplay between the sexes. Just as moden psychologists and sex therapists have encouraged us to consider the entire sex act as important, the Taoists considered the whole process as symbolic of universal interrelationship. Paradoxically though, the "selfish" Taoist lover is just the opposite of what we might call selfish in our modern society.

A balanced Taoist magician has an attitude of "equal exchange," while the negative or neurotic Taoist is out for all he can gain personally. He views sex as a struggle or contest. The selfish attitude of using partners to gain immortality consists of inducing one's sex partner to as many orgasms as possible while conserving one's own juices. Western society, on the other hand, considers a lover selfish who values his own orgasms over mutual pleasure.

Taoists practiced sex as a form of meditation which could continue for several days. In order to maintain their vigor, they sought to remain in a state of philosophical calm. By not striving and by remaining detached and cool, they used their concentration to increase sensitivity in every part of the body. This awakened the most subtle sensations in a slowly unfolding process.

Sex with totally awakened consciousness of the "now" can be enjoyed as an end in itself. Since the partner who is first to reach orgasm provides the other with an abundance of life force, sex may be seen as a mock battle in which the "opponents" compete to see who can induce the other to climax. Rather than approaching this as a matter of survival, we could view it as refreshing recreational sex play. Even though it is an arbitrary attitude, in the West orgasm is considered the supreme goal and reward of sex. Aside from certain magical practices (see damiana), failure to experience sexual release is considered harmful and neurotic. But this attitude contains a cultural bias.

We have become obsessed with "achieving" orgasms, the more the better. We may have lost something by paying little attention to the quality of the experience. An evening of "Taoist lovemaking" might restore some specialness to your relationship. Incorporate some subtle nuances by maximizing body contact with your partner while minimizing leaking of vital fluids. If the partners attempt to complement and harmonize with one another, both will be nourished. When the desire for orgasm is so strong it cannot be resisted, we may submit, and then revive ourselves by sipping some ginseng tea!

Masters of the more advanced Taoist techniques delved into the problem of not wasting their essences, devising ways to prolong pleasure and stave off release. As "physicians" they prescribed herbs and medicines to restore virility. Taoist sages also considered what sexual positions were most effective as cures for specific ailments.

Note of Caution: *Ginseng is available in most health-food stores for anyone wanting to be "mitogenically" radiated and/or sexually inspired. Good grades of ginseng can be purchased for as little as $5.00 per ounce, but take care not to purchase the low-quality Japanese varieties (common in the market). All potent grades of ginseng are comparatively expensive.*

Most Chinese herbalists divide ginseng into at least four grades. The most expensive is the wild Tung Pei, one ounce of roots bringing more than $5,500. Small roots weigh about one gram and are sold for $100.

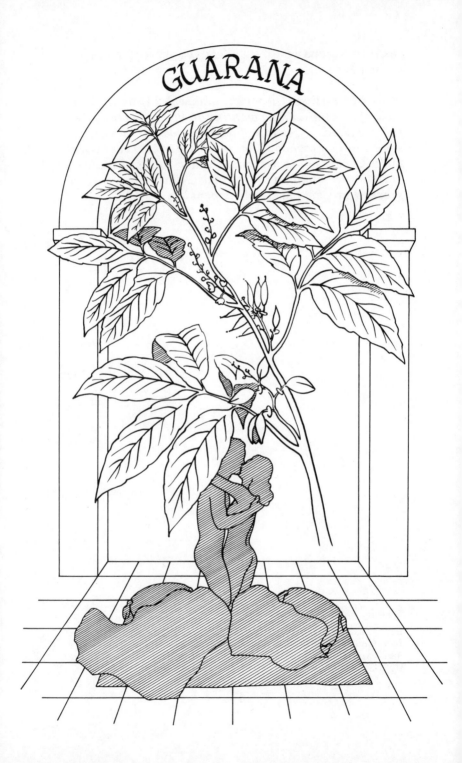

Guarana

Family: Sapindaceae (Soapberry).

Botanical Name: *Paullinia cupana.*

Synonyms: Panela supana, Brazilian cocoa, uabano.

Geographical Location: South America, particularly northern and western Brazil; also some parts of Venezuela.

Habitat: South American tropical jungles in the Amazon.

Botanical Description: A climbing shrub with divided compounded leaves. The flowers are yellow in an open cluster. The three-celled capsuled fruit contains a seed resembling small horse chestnuts in each of the three cells. The fresh seeds are flesh colored and are easily separated from the fruit after drying. The seeds are washed and then roasted for six hours before use.

History: Guarana was first used by the Quaramis, a tribe of South American Indians, for bowel complaints. It was also used by Brazilian miners as a preventative for diseases but was mainly used as a refreshing beverage. It is now used as a main ingredient in a favorite diet beverage in Brazil.

Natives in the same Amazon basin region carry long rods of hardened guarana powder and grate it whenever they need a substitute for food. They can travel for two or even three days without eating if they have this precious rod to nibble on. Usually taken in powdered form, these seeds seem also somewhat aphrodisiac, due primarily to the large amounts of guaranine, a little-understood oil that is slightly hallucinogenic. (Guarana is now used in a number of over-the-counter appetite suppressants.)

Chemistry: Guarana falls in the methylated purine group containing 5 percent caffeine, or three times as much as in normal coffee. Guarana is considered the strongest naturally occurring methylxanthine. It has the same chemical composition as caffeine, theine, and cocaine, and the same physiological action.

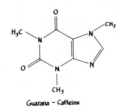

Guarana – Caffeine

Other methylated purines are:

a) Coffee *(Coffea arabica)* - An Arabian bush; bean contains 1 to 2 percent caffeine.

b) Tea *(Camelia theca)* - An Asian bush; leaves contain 2 to 4 percent caffeine, with theobromine and theophylline.

c) Cacao *(Theobroma cacao)* - Aztec, chocolate; beans contain 2 percent theobromine and traces of caffeine and theophylline.

44

d) Mate' (Ilex paraguyensis) - A South American bush; leaves contain 2 to 3 percent caffeine.

e) Kola *(Cola nitida)* - An African tree; nut contains 3 percent caffeine.

Primary Effects: Stimulant. Quickens perceptions and wakefulness, slows the pulse, impairs the appetite, and can be used for long drives or long work hours.

Preparation: Powder guarana seed with a mortar and pestle or coffee grinder. Prepared like coffee, the grounds can be used several times. Two nuts are recommended per cup. The powder can also be put in 00 capsules if the brewed flavor is undesirable.

Ritual Use: Since guarana is a stimulant, it can make us seem more inspired or interesting in both conversation and appearance. Drink some before that "heavy date" or big event to perk up your spirits and your looks.

From the most ancient times, cosmetics and ornaments have played a major role in sexual ritual as well as in simple courting. The application of make-up can become a personal encounter between the self that one is at the moment and the self that one wishes to project. Remember, the mirror is one of the time-honored symbols of Aphrodite. Guarana is an excellent mood elevator during one's ritual before a mirror since most applications of make-up take time and patience.

Before the advent of our modern "muscle shirts" and lingerie, many mystical rites made use of specific make-up and ornaments to stimulate particular sentiments. The importance of cosmetics in the present day can be gauged by their enormous worldwide sales. Tantric rites specify body make-up and jewelry for aesthetic, psychological, symbolic, and even physiological effects. For example, heavy earrings rubbing on the neck create a continual low-level stimulation thought to enhance arousal or sensuality in the wearer.

For Tantric rites of sex magic, the body is bathed

and lightly oiled and then dusted all over with ashes (a modern equivalent might be a scented dusting powder). Wood ash contains valuable trace minerals that are easily absorbed through the skin. Pure ash from selected hardwoods (such as oak) has an invigorating and insulating effect on the body and is said to protect it against psychic disturbances.

Once the wood ash is applied, exact marks (usually groups of three parallel lines) are made on the lower legs, thighs, forearms, upper arms, between the sexual region and the navel, across the navel, in the middle of the chest, and on the throat and the forehead. These are made with a powder or ointment from crushed sandalwood, herbs, cereal grains, and intoxicating ingredients. There is no doubt some profound symbology for the tantrics in these marks, but by and large they are merely deemed attractive as are the tattoos and odd deformations of the body in various other cultures of the world.

The most common custom is for the man to look handsome, using ash and marks, while the woman should look seductive and sensual, using face make-up and with other parts of the body colored red, which is considered an exciting color. The color red is known to effectively stimulate the male sex centers and is one reason for its use in so many facial cosmetics and in sexually appealing clothing. One's inherent sexual potential is activated by the careful and dramatic use of make-up. A virile-looking man and a seductive woman symbolize the union of male aggressive energy with female receptivity.

In Tantric ritual, especially during sex magic, a woman is expected to wear her most symbolic jewelry. When arrayed with full ornamentation, a beautiful woman is able to excite and stimulate any man. You should try to make use of cosmetics and jewelry whenever possible. This will enhance your natural charms and increase aesthetic delight.

Note of Caution: *Long-term or excessive use of guarana alters the blood sugar. This will cause nervousness, insomnia, and possible psychic habituation. Use supplements to replace B vitamins and calm the nerves.*

Guarana can also be used as a tonic nervine against hangovers, menstrual headaches, and neuralgia.

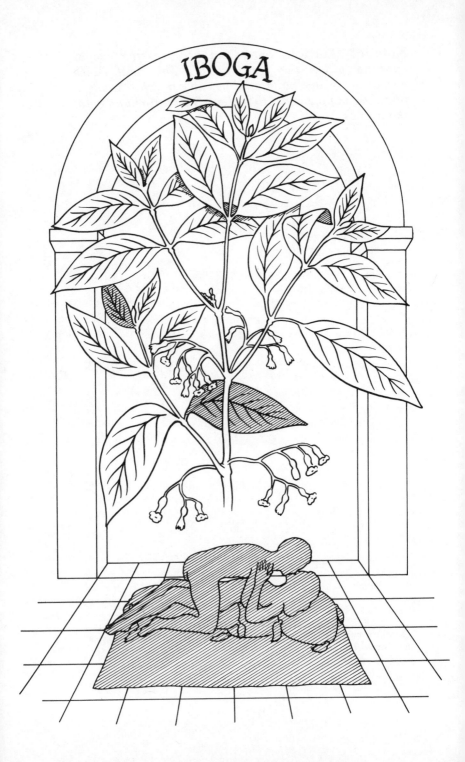

*A powerful stimulant and hallucinogen
for Sex Magic rituals*

Iboga'

Family: Apocynaceae.

Botanical Name: *Tabernanthe iboga* B.

Synonyms: None.

Geographical Location: Gabon and the surrounding parts of the Republic of the Congo; also, a large area of Zaire. It is now also cultivated in West Africa beyond its natural range.

Habitat: Forest and jungle.

Botanical Description: It is a shrub 3 to 6 feet tall, with leaves that are lanceolate, opposite, and up to 3 inches long. The roots are robust and branched. The flowers are white spotted with pink and contorted in bud. The fruit is a berry with seeds that have fleshy ruminate albumen. The root is yellowish.

History: The powdered bark (especially the root bark) of the iboga' forest shrub is consumed by the natives of Gabon and part of the Congo in the initiation rites of a number of secret societies. The most famous of these societies is the *Bwiti* or *Bouiti,* where the drug has far-reaching social effects. Sorcerers, for example, take the drug before seeking information from the spirit world, and cult leaders eat iboga' root for a whole day before asking advice from dead ancestors.

It is also chewed before the lion hunt. The drug enables the hunter to remain awake while standing motionless for as long as forty-eight hours. In this position he patiently waits for the lion to cross his path—or so the story goes.

The Bwiti, an African secret society, demand from its applicants that before they can be admitted as members they must have seen their holy god plant *Bwiti* in their visions. For the initiation ceremony, a potion containing large quantities of the iboga' root is taken.

The drug is also consumed by those who believe it can reveal objects *(ogbanje)* reputedly buried by individuals subjected to the intoxicant during their former lives. Among natives, it has for centuries been considered a powerful aphrodisiac and stimulant, reportedly doubling muscular strength and enabling hunters to stay motionless for hours while stalking game.

In the Bwiti mythology the Creator God dismembered a pigmy and planted his parts in the forest. His wife discovered that iboga' plants had risen from her husband's flesh. She was instructed by the Creator God to eat of their roots so that she might once more communicate with the spirit of her dead husband and moreover have a knowledge of the supernatural. From that time hence the Bwiti have venerated this iboga' plant and partake of its flesh by chewing on the root cortex.

When the French occupied that area of equatorial Africa, they sent root cortex back to France. Their chemists made a crude extract which they sold as *Lambarence. Lambarence* was used in western Europe at the beginning of this century as a reputed cure-all, being applied to diseases from neurasthenia to syphilis. The French could also not ignore what the Bwiti tradition said concerning the aphrodisiac properties of the root.

Occasionally, other plants (sometimes as many as ten), are taken with iboga'. One of the interesting additives is the euphorbiaceous *Alchornea floribunda,* known in Liberia, Nigeria, and Uganda as *niando.* The root bark of this shrub of the spurge family is macerated in palm or banana wine and drunk for its stimulating influence on the libido. Studies show that the roots and seeds of this plant contain yohimbine, making this combination of niando and iboga' dangerous since it forms an MAO inhibitor.

Monamine oxidase (MAO) is an enzyme that causes the breakdown of certain chemical messengers (neurotransmitters) in the neurons of the human brain. MAO inhibitors reduce the degradations of these substances, markedly increasing their concentrations. This can produce a hypotensive crisis with symptoms that include breathing difficulties, heart palpitations, chills, and a sharp drop in blood pressure. Other substances that exaggerate this reaction are tricyclic antidepressant drugs, alcohol, amphetamines, avocados, unripe bananas, and ripe cheeses.

Chemistry: Six percent of the dried roots contain twelve closely related indoles, the principle one being ibogaine. Ibogaine seems to be mainly responsible for the psychopharmacological effects of the crude drug. These effects may be divided into three parts:

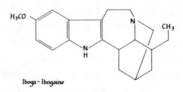

Iboga - Ibogaine

1. Inhibition of cholinesterase, causing hypotension and stimulation of digestion and appetite.

51

2. Strong central nervous system stimulation, leading in toxic doses to convulsions, paralysis, and arrest of respiration.

3. Visual and other hallucinations that are sometimes associated with severe anxiety and apprehension.

Primary Effects: With doses of 300 mg dried root bark powder, many experience slight nausea, dizziness, and a lack of muscular control or coordination. There are also some changes in perception. Visual imagery is vivid behind closed eyes, and heightened empathy provides real insight into self and relationships.

Preparation: Capsulate 1 gram dried and powdered iboga' root into 00 capsules. This is the amount that can be taken by someone already experienced in the use of iboga'. First-time experimenters should begin by taking 200 mg or 1/5 the normal dosage. Do not take it with other drugs or alcohol, and take it on an empty stomach. Some will feel nausea, and some may vomit or experience lack of muscular coordination. Some of this discomfort can be eliminated by fasting for 18 hours before ingesting it and by taking 2 to 3 dramamine (air sickness pills) 1 hour before ingestion of iboga' powder.

Ritual Use: Most of the original concepts of sex, as it relates to magic, are from the earlier eastern traditions of Tantric Buddhism. Tantric cults held that sex contained an energy that could change the physical world. The first use of sex within the rituals of western traditions of magic began with the *Ordo Templi Orientis* (O.T.O.), an 800-year old Masonic order headquartered in Germany. Its members practiced a form of alchemy, a process of psychic and physical transformation.

Coniunctio is an alchemical term symbolizing the unification of opposites. When the opposites to be united are the masculine consciousness and the feminine unconsciousness, the union is termed the royal marriage. This royal marriage is a transcendent symbol of the self and embodies psychic totality, or wholeness.

This psycho-sexual energy is the principal element behind contemporary western magic today. In the East, it is known as kundalini, or the serpent power. It is the single strongest emotion alterant available, channeling sexual energy into a process of self-development. It is the foundation of Tantra.

Sex magic is described metaphorically in alchemical terms in Israel Regardie's classic on western magic, *The Tree of Life* (Chapter 16). He learned of sex magic in his work with the occult group known as The Golden Dawn and as a colleague of Aleister Crowley, who headed the Ordo Templi Orientis during his later years. O.T.O. rites reflect their ancestry in Tantric Buddhism and contain great power. Aleister Crowley expounded his complete formula for sex magic in both *Liber Samekh* and *Liber Aleph, The Book of Wisdom or Folly* (page 86). Restated in more common terms, it involves the following steps (presupposed are active magical pathworking, an oath, banishing rites, and so on.)

1. *Discover your true will.* What is the purpose of this magical operation? Is it absolutely necessary and desirable? Are you at a psychological impasse? Is your personality stable or unstable? Do not seek to actualize your lower desires with sex magic. Its proper application is personal transformation.

2. *Personify your intent by naming it.* Concoct an imagined form to express your will by using appropriate symbolism. For example, if your desire is for a balanced personality picture yourself *being* that in nascent form.

3. *Purify and consecrate this entity.* Make sure it is a pure archetypal form uncontaminated by your complexes and prejudices. As a "child" it is all potential. This is the phase of generating desire through foreplay

while constantly keeping the attention on the purpose of the magical operation.

4. *Visualize the image of the magical child upon entry.* This visualization might be the actualization of your own potential or a vision of yourself in the future. The union of opposites offers the "child" a vehicle for manifestation once the gestation period is full. There is a synergetic effect here as both partners contemplate the creation of the child. Their visualizations should be as identical as possible for the best results. This invocation creates a current of force or psychological energy to help manifest your will.

5. *Consummate the marriage with a golden ring.* This is a euphemism for the climax or orgasm. This moment just before orgasm is a very open, oceanic psychological state and a potent time for reprogramming the subconscious. You can change yourself now, just as habits can be altered with autohypnosis. Careful control of the attention at this moment is vital to success. Don't let the thoughts wander at this time even in regular sexual relations, as the thought held at this moment *tends to manifest!*

6. *Consume the eucharist (consecrated substance).* The power of the sexual act has been transferred to a material body symbolized by the mingled fluids of the partners. Eating the sexual fluids means that one assimilates and digests, or integrates, the qualities represented by the "Magical Child" as the union of opposites. It is a part of oneself, united with its opposite and made one's self again. It is love reborn.

There are greater and lesser forms of *coniunctio* in the process of psychological transformation. In the early stages comes the union with the shadow. This signifies the reunion of mind and body. This heals our Cartesian duality, or the cultural mind-body split. Later comes the reunification with anima/animus (our

54

contrasexual nature), then union with the higher self. This final *coniunctio* produces spiritual rebirth in an experience of the "one world," where body, soul, and spirit are reunited.

One must be extremely careful in employing sex magic! The criteria for all other rituals of transformation apply, including "is this absolutely necessary?" Usually this is not the case, and the impulsive aspirant bites off more than he can chew. Literal practice of sex magic on the physical plane might represent a gross misunderstanding of what should be an internal psychological process. Be careful not to confuse the discrete planes of awareness that include the physical, emotional, psychological, and spiritual levels of meaning.

Remember that you will get what you ask for (i.e., the bud-will), but you may get a great deal you had not bargained for in karmic repercussions and unforeseen consequences!

Note of Caution: *Normal amounts may cause nausea, vomiting, and circulatory disturbances. Convulsions, paralysis, and respiratory collapse occur with overdoses. Do not use it if you are prone to low blood pressure or are in fragile health. Do not combine with foods that promote the formation of MAO inhibitors.*

Iboga' is one of the plants that animals eat to get high. Gorillas, porcupines, and wild boars in Gabon and the northern Congo are said to favor it. Natives say wild boars dig up and eat the roots, "only to go into a wild frenzy of jumping around, perhaps fleeing from frightening visions."

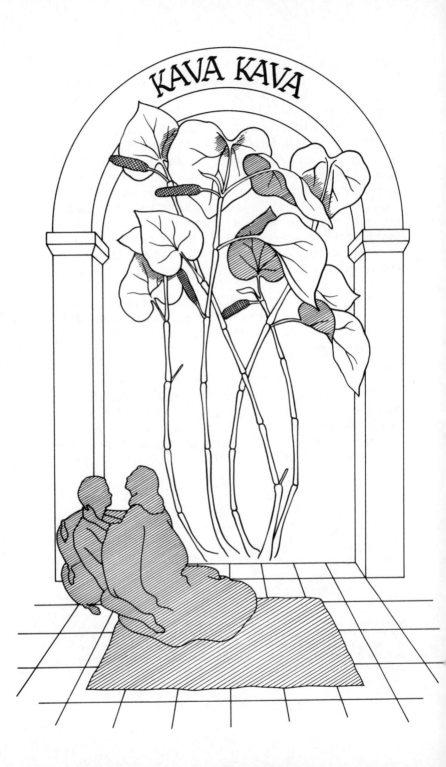

*An herb from Fiji for Dharana—
control of thought*

Kava Kava

Family: Piperceae (Pepper).

Botanical Description: *Piper methysticum* Forst.

Synonyms: Kowa, awa, yaona, kowa kowa, wati, ava, ava pepper, intoxicating pepper.

Geographical Location: Polynesia, Sandwich Islands, South Sea Islands.

Habitat: Grows best up to 1,000 feet above sea level in cool, moist highlands or wet forests. It will grow densely to 20 feet where summer temperatures are between 80 and 90°F if it has sufficient sunlight.

Botanical Description: An indigenous shrub several feet high with heart-shaped leaves and very short spikes arising from the base of leaf stems that are densely covered with flowers. The stem is dictiotomous, that is, two-forked, with spots. The upper rhyzome is the part of the plant that is used and is starchy with a faint pleasant odor and a pungent, bitter taste.

Five varieties are cultivated in Fiji, three white and two black. The white varieties are considered the best sources, but mature one year later than the black. The black varieties are preferred for the commerical crop.

History: Kava kava has a history of religious and spiritual implications in the affairs of men. An excellent legend, summarizing man's relationship to the sun, sky, water, and earth is given in *The Magical and Ritual Use of Herbs* (Destiny Books). This alchemical marriage of fire, wind, water, and earth is related to the spiritual "other" part of the soul, or "divine being" part of the mortal self.

Kava's history and chemistry indicate that its euphoric qualities are best shared with special guests (or even lovers) because the narcotic effects stimulate the "feeling" centers. Warm emotions are generated toward those involved, and as a consequence, kava kava has been used as a sacrament for welcoming special guests and friends.

Chemistry: Active components in kava kava are six resinous alpha pyrones: kawain ($C_{14}H_{14}O_3$), dihydrokawain, methysticin ($C_{15}H_{14}O_5$), dihydromethysticin, yangonin ($C_{15}H_{14}O_3$), and dihyroyangonin. None of these are water soluble except when emulsified. They are soluble in alcohol, oils, and other fat solvents (including gastric juices).

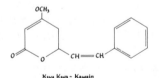

Kava Kava - Kawain

Primary Effects: Small amounts produce euphoria; larger amounts produce extreme relaxation, lethargy of the lower limbs and, eventually, sleep. It does not impair mental alertness. There are often visual and auditory hallucinations that last from two to three hours with no hangover. Kava kava is similar to marijuana in that the effects are fairly subtle and not noticed when used for the first several times. As a narcotic kava kava later produces numbing of the mouth, a numbing similar to that produced by cocaine.

Preparation: The part of the kava kava plant just below the surface of the ground reaches a 3 to 5 inch thickness in 2 to 4 years. After 6 years, the root will weigh as much as 20 pounds, and after 20 years, 100 pounds. After harvesting, the root stocks are scraped, cut into pieces, and dried in the sun on platforms.

Traditionally the root was made into a tea. With its water-soluble components released, it acted as a mild stimulant and tonic. If the material is first chewed, then spit into a bowl and mixed with coconut milk, more powerful resins resembling narcotics are released in emulsion. For maximum effect, mix 1 ounce of kava kava with 10 ounces of water (or coconut milk), 2 tablespoons of coconut or olive oil, and 1 tablespoon of lecithin. Blend until the liquid takes on a milky appearance. This amount serves 1 to 2 persons.

Resins may be extracted with isopropyl (rubbing) alcohol in a heated bath. The solvent is removed by evaporation. Redissolve in just enough warmed brandy. rum, vodka, or honey. This is a more potent method because alcohol swiftly carries the resins into the body's system.

Ritual Use: Within the sex magic rituals of Tantric yoga there is a need to control thought and to visualize. The yoga of thought control is called *Dharana,* or concentration. Visualization is known as *Dhyan.* Both hold the mind one pointedly.

When our minds try to concentrate (perhaps through repetition of a word), our attention is repeatedly diverted from our subject of meditation. *Dharana* develops the ability to concentrate on one subject. Kava kava is an excellent aphrodisiac that can be used to assist in this exercise to develop mental images and thoughts. When the body is comfortably alert, attention may be concentrated on a mental exercise or visualization for an uninterrupted period of time. If the mind diverges from the subject, gently return to the meditation as often as necessary.

Fixing the attention is the only way of stilling the senses and the mind in this yoga of "self-absorption." One's attention becomes focused internally; the thoughts are restrained and the senses don't flow out into the world. This creates bliss.

In Tantra both inner and outer pleasures are combined. First, internal concentration is perfected so that when meditation is combined with the pleasures of the sex act the personality does not become submerged in lower desires. The sense pleasures employed in Tantra are of five classes: 1) beautiful forms and colors that attract the eyes; 2) enchanting sounds or melodies for the ears; 3) delectable foods to captivate the palate; 4) fragrant scents; and 5) pleasing physical sensations from direct contact. Concentrating on any of our sense perceptions collects the wandering mind at a focal point.

Eastern yogis also practice Dharana on master souls, or external objects like the sun, moon, and planets. One might also contemplate the internal centers, or chakras. It is also possible to contemplate one's self to learn the power of pure cognition without resorting to the aid of the senses or outer reality. This is known as the process of self-realization and creates the emergence of several occult powers as its byproduct. In Dharana these abilities are not as important as perfecting the ability to still the mind.

There are five distinct levels of concentration of attention. In the first, the mind wanders and thoughts are continually dispersed and scattered. The second level is a condition of lethargy, confusion, and forgetfulness. At the third level the mind develops intermittent stability. The attention collects momentarily and then disperses. Finally, the attention is fixed in its purpose, which leads to a mind that is disciplined and able to concentrate at will.

The following is an important set of exercises in Dharana.

1. Constrain the mind to concentrate upon a single, simple imagined object. The five tatwas, which correspond to each element, are useful for this purpose: a yellow square—earth *(Prithiva)*, a red triangle—fire or light *(Tejas)*, a silver crescent—water *(Apas)*, a blue disk—air *(Vayu)*, and a black oval—spirit *(Akasa)*.

2. Once you can readily concentrate on these simple forms, proceed to a combination of simple objects. For example, try to concentrate on a black oval within a yellow square or a silver crescent within the black oval.

3. When you are successful with the second stage, proceed to visualize simple moving objects, such as a pendulum swinging or a wheel revolving. Do not attempt to picture living objects at this point.

4. Proceed to a combination of moving objects. Examples might include pulleys and gears or pistons. You might even make up your own "Rube Goldberg" contraption to illustrate the laws of cause and effect. The ultimate aim here is the vision of the "machinery of the universe."

During these practices the mind must be alert and absolutely confined to the object decided upon. No other thought must be allowed to intrude upon consciousness. The moving systems must be regular and harmonious.

Carefully note the duration of the experiments, the number and nature of the intruding thoughts, the tendency of the object itself to depart from the course laid out for it, and any other phenomena that may present themselves. It is very important to avoid overstrain.

5. Proceed to imagine living objects such as a woman. It is best to visualize a person who is known and respected. This prepares us to concentrate on the visualization of our Tantric partner as a symbolic representative of divine universal forces.

6. In the intervals of these experiments you may try to imagine the objects of the other senses and concentrate upon them. For example, try to remember the taste of your favorite delicacy, the scent of your favorite flower or perfume, the feeling of velvet or soft skin, the sound of a tinkling bell or rushing waterfall.

7. Endeavor finally to shut out all objects of any of the senses, and prevent all thoughts from arising in your mind. To aid this, gather your attention in the center behind the eyes known as the third eye, Ajna Chakra, or the pituitary-pineal gland area of the brain. When you feel you have attained some success in these practices, you are probably ready to apply them in a formal Tantric sex magic ritual.

Each type of exercise can be employed to enhance your ritual experience. For example, you might choose to adorn your forehead with one of the tatwas or a combination of tatwas symbolizing your elemental qualities. One might approach the rite with a pervasive feeling of one's place in the great cosmic plan, which is in the constant flux of relative motion. When you merge with your partner, you *are* the divine forces of Shiva and Shakti locked in eternal embrace. Thus spirit and matter create the universe. Then one becomes a wave in the ocean of pure consciousness as the senses are transcended.

Note of Caution: *Continual chewing of kava kava will eventually destroy tooth enamel. Constant and excessive use of the fresh root with alcohol can become habit forming after several months, resulting in yellowing of the skin, bloodshot and weak eyes, emaciation, diarrhea, rashes, and scaly, ulcerous skin. When discontinued, these symptoms will disappear within two weeks.*

Kawain chemistry also has surface anesthetic properties similar to cocaine alkaloids. In the islands, kava kava leaves are often applied to cuts and bruises to prevent infection and to promote healing. The kava kava pyrones have antibacterial properties that act against gonococcus and coli bacilli.

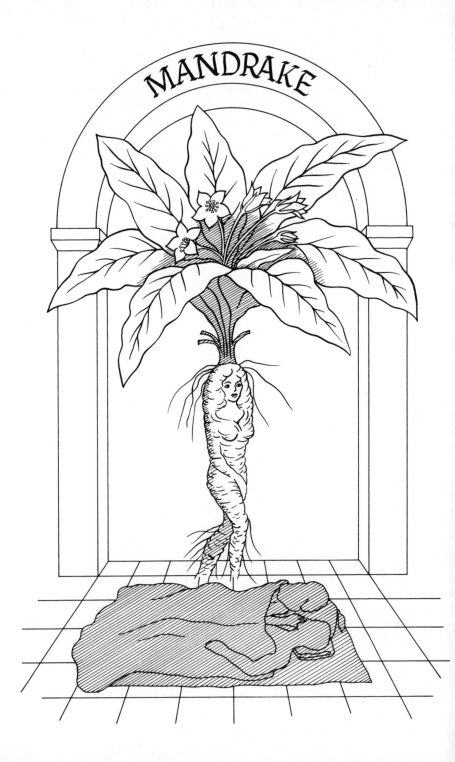

An aphrodisiac to aid conception and fertility and allegedly reverse sterility

Mandrake

Family: Solanaceae (Potatoe).

Botanical Name: *Mandragora officianarum.*

Synonyms: Satan's Apple, mandragora, love apple, Circe's plant, *Dudaim.*

Geographical Location: Native to Southern Europe, especially around the Mediterranean regions of Greece and Rome. It should not be confused with *Podophyllum peltatum,* or May apple, which grows in the United States.

Habitat: Uncultivated fields and stony wastelands. It can be cultivated in gardens if given a warm situation; it does not survive severe winters.

Botanical Description: It has a large brown root (like a parsnip), running 3 to 4 feet into the ground. The root is thick and is frequently forked like two legs. It has a short stem topped by ovate leaves. Its fruit consists of fleshy berries of an orange color. A species of mandrake, *Mandragora autumnalis,* flowers in winter on the island of Rhodes with beautiful mauve and

65

mauve-white blossoms. The fruit, the golden-red love apple, ripens in May.

History: The best known of all the aphrodisiacs of the ancient world was the mandrake or mandragora, a purple-flowered tuber with roots that often resembled the human body. The earliest reflection of the belief in the value of mandrake as an aphrodisiac and as an aid to conception is in the biblical passage

"And Reuban went in the days of wheat harvest, and found mandrakes in the field, and brought them unto his mother Leah. Then Rachel said to Leah, 'Give me, I pray thee, of thy son's mandrakes.'

And she said unto her, 'Is it a small matter that thou hast taken my husband? And wouldst thou take away my son's mandrakes also?

And Rachel said, 'Therefore he shall lie with thee tonight for thy son's mandrakes.

And Jacob came out of the field in the evening, and Leah went out to meet him, and said, 'Thou must come in unto me; for surely I have hired thee with my son's mandrakes.' And he lay with her that night

And God harkened unto Leah, and she conceived and bore Jacob the fifth son."

GENESIS 30:14-17

There is only one more reference to the mandrake in the *Old Testament:*

"The mandrakes give a smell, and at our gates are all manner of pleasant fruits, new and old, which I have laid up for thee, O my beloved."

SONG OF SOLOMON 7:13

The Hebrew word *Dudaim* has been translated in the *Song of Solomon* as "mandrake." The word *Dudaim* indicates a fruit with a sweet and agreeable odor much in demand by the male sex. The word is probably derived from *Dudim* (the pleasure of love) and has been translated as "apples." It was also valued in ancient Greece and Rome for its narcotic properties and was used as a surgical anesthetic.

A fable originating sometime in second-century Rome warns that whoever pulled a mandrake out of the ground would suffer the dire consequences of the deed. The demon who inhabited the root would be aroused and the sounds of its piercing shrieks of agony would be so horrible that they would kill the harvester on the spot. The ritual goes on to say that if one drew three circles around the plant with the tip of a willow wand and tied a black thread from the plant to the collar of a white dog, one would be safe from the demon's spell as the animal pulled it from the ground.

The roots of mandrake were supposed to bear a resemblance to the human form. Magically speaking, there are male and female mandrakes. The female form, its roots forked and looking like a pair of human legs, is the most sought after. The male, on the other hand, has a single root. It was the "female" form that was carved in the Middle Ages (in Germany and France) into mannikins. It was believed that they brought good luck and wealth.

Chemistry: Principle active components are scopolomine (hyoscine), atropine, hyosyamine, and mandragorine. These tropanes are all parasympathetic depressants. The chemistry of mandrake is similar to that of datura and is exceptionally rich in mandragorine, a powerful narcotic and hypnotic ($C_{17}H_{27}O_3N$).

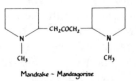

Mandrake ~ Mandragorine

Primary Effects: Parasympathetic depressant. Hallucinogen and hypnotic. Most hypnotics produce low alphoid and spindal alpha brain-wave activity, similar to those found in REM sleep, or the dreaming state. This rhythm does not allow deep sleep to occur although it does lower brain patterns into a dreamy visionary mode, known in magic as an experience of the astral plane.

Preparation: The root is powdered and small quantities are placed in wine, usually using less than 30 grains of the root. Both the fruit and the roots were used as ingredients in "flying ointments," psychedelic preparations allegedly used by fifteenth-century witches for flying on their brooms in astral projection.

Ritual Use: Mandrake is primarily considered as an aphrodisiac because of its resemblance to the human figure. Of the two distinct types of love magic, the first is the general charm or medicine which allegedly "works" on anyone and which is selected because of its distinctive appearance, shape, taste, or easily recognized symbolism. This type is seen, for instance, in the most highly valued ginsengs (also resembling the human form) or in the likeness of the female organs to the oyster.

The fact that mandrake is almost an anaphrodisiac because of its parasympathetic depressant chemistry leads one to consider using it for sexual fantasies rather than for physical activity. It is conducive to an astral fantasy and has a tradition of use in this manner. This is the origin of the famous stories about witches flying on their broomsticks to attend orgies at their Sabbats. They experienced astral journeys in which their repressed sexuality came vividly to life. These were considered evil since sex was considered "Satanic."

Today mandrake is not considered demonic, and sex is not Satanic. Because it does not allow deep sleep states to occur, mandrake is well-suited to those altered states in which lucid or "waking dreams" occur very near consciousness. Too often we are unaware of our inner feelings, unaware of the hidden aspects of our personalities, and out of touch with our unconscious emotions. In this sense we are much like medieval people in our personal psychologies.

We can get in touch with ourselves and some of our deepest feelings by using our dreams. When seen on this level, dreams can reveal a person's basic feelings, values, philosophy, and methods of coping with emotional problems. The appearance of symbols is individual and personal, depending on one's life experience. Content includes the *mood* of the dream and the emotions felt while dreaming. A sexual "waking dream" can be pre-programmed if one's mood and concentration remain constant after imbibing the mandrake.

Dream symbols express and extend our waking thoughts rather than disguise them to protect us. Training yourself to remember and use your dreams can be a pleasant and helpful day-to-day exercise and should not be distorted into an agonizing probing for sin and guilt. Exposing problems that we may have refused to accept consciously can lead to positive, corrective action. It can lead to the recognition of emotions that we have tried to submerge, eventually motivating us to accept, or perhaps even control or channel them.

When taken in small doses, mandrake will produce a light, sleep-like trance with very lucid dreams. The effects last for several hours. Immediately upon awakening, whether in the middle of the night or in the morning, try to recapture the dream you were having.

Write down a summary that includes both its content and mood. Think about what your emotions were during the dream and what your feelings about it are now that you are awake.

Don't worry about any deep probing of symbolism for the first dream; simply enjoy the fact that you caught it. If you wish to reflect on its content, do so, but the purpose of the first exercise is simply to experience the fact that you are now touching a part of yourself that you have probably paid little attention to until now. All increases in self-awareness or understanding make us better lovers. The mandrake keeps your consciousness close enough to the surface that the contact between the conscious and subconscious selves is quite real in experience.

Note of Caution: *Mandrake can be detrimental to the heart because of the tropanes. A tolerance is built up to the tropanes in the parasympathetic system; thus more mandrake is required to achieve the same "effects." This is* not *true with the effects on the heart, and severe damage may occur. It is extremely toxic.*

Mandrake can be made into extracts with ethyl alcohol. A smoke can then be prepared by dipping tobacco or herbal cigarettes into the extract and letting them air dry.

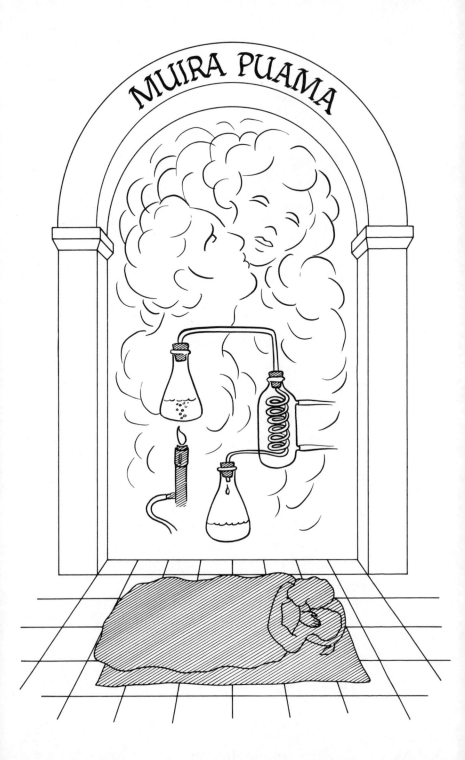

Muira Puama

Family: Olacaceae.

Botanical Name: *Liriosma ovata.*

Synonyms: None.

Geographical Location: In the region around the Amazon and Orinoco Basin of Brazil.

Habitat: Forests and jungles.

Botanical Description: A small tree, 6 to 12 feet tall. The roots and bark are slightly pink and resemble madrone.

History: The natives of the Amazon and Orinoco Basin chew the bark or boil the roots and bark to make a potent beverage. Their standard preparation is to boil 2 to 4 tablespoons of the shaved wood for about 15 minutes in 1 pint of water. Each would drink one cup of the strained liquid 1 to 2 hours before coitus.

Chemistry: It contains an unidentified resin with strong stimulating effects upon the central nervous system and libido. This resin is not water soluble and thus, boiling it in water and ingesting it via the stomach is not the most efficient way to take it.

Primary Effects: Chills up and down the spine after two hours of ingesting the raw herb in capsules, similar in physical effects to yohimbe bark. Although the effects are more subtle than yohimbe, more than 70 percent of the people who have used this bark/root do feel its effects.

Preparation: It is better to extract 4 tablespoons of the muira-puama bark powder into 1/2 pint of boiling vodka for 15 minutes. Strain while still hot and drink 1 or 2 cordial glasses about 1 hour before coitus.

The resin can be extracted by immersing in hot isopropanol (or any other) alcohol. Strain the mixture and evaporate the solvent in a double boiler or heat bath. The remaining resin is then gathered and refrigerated. One pellet about the size of a pea can be placed in the mouth one and a half hours before coitus and should be allowed to dissolve in the saliva before it is swallowed.

Some have even smoked the bark, but the smoke is excessively harsh. It is unpleasant to chew because wood splinters tend to catch in the throat. The powder is often capsulized, but again, it is poorly assimilated in the stomach because of the resin's suspension in the water and digestive juices.

Ritual Use: Muira-puama is useful for reflection or self-evaluation. Understanding our patterns of behavior can be an important step in self-development. Self-understanding makes us more at ease with ourselves and others. Muira-puama enhances sensuality as well as sexuality. There are various styles of love and lovers in the world. What kind of lover are you? When we become excited, we express more of our innate style.

A knowledge of various categories of love and lovers is useful to provide depth of meaning in the sexual encounter. Through a knowledge of types, we can learn to anticipate what to expect, both from ourselves and others. Characteristic patterns, or roles, develop in all human relationships. An understanding of these patterns provides a useful orientation in defining the interplay between love and sex. Sip your cordial and contemplate on the following.

The Greeks distinguished three kinds of love relationships, *eros, philia,* and *agape.*

Eros, according to the philosophers, was a personal, emotional, passionate love. It could include physical attraction but could also arise from internal psychological need. The sexual component has become dominant in our contemporary consciousness to the point that "erotic" now means "sexual."

Philia implies brotherly/sisterly love and is reflected in the name of the city of Philadelphia, the City of Brotherly Love. This includes companionship and nonsexual affection and caring, and is today referred to as platonic love. This is the affection of co-workers who share interests in common. This kind of love also extends to nonhuman forms of life and even inanimate objects. For example, some people love animals, plants, rocks, or their shiny new car or silky dress.

Agape is an exalted form of spiritual, or cosmic love. It is an all-embracing feeling of unity that is totally nonexclusive. It culminates in a mystical experience of oneness with all of life. This kind of love was also known as *caritas* in Latin and was later translated as "charity" in several English versions of the Bible. It is exemplified in the love of the devotee for the teacher and the teacher's compassion for the disciple.

In the cultural worlds of Rome and the Christian Middle Ages, *eros* became *amor,* a romantic love of courting, being in love for "love's sake." It became less lusty and physical. Physical desires became *libido* in Latin, eventually being adapted by Sigmund Freud as the single term for the primal energy, which he recognized as sexual in nature. *Caritas* became a religious concept; it was the love of God for man.

The Eastern view of the types of love is characterized in a traditional Indian formulation known as *The Five Stages of Love*. It is through these stages that a devotee has to pass in his or her relationship to the Divine Being within the self.

The First Stage: The first criteria consists of absolute loving obedience, like that of a servant for the master.

The Second Stage: This stage of love takes the form of friendship, implying a relationship between peers. We assume a first-name basis with the characters of our inner drama of transformation.

The Third Stage: This phase is maternal in quality. The devotee cultivates and nourishes the divine child within.

The Fourth Stage: One behaves as a spouse; the union between two individuals is both physical and spiritual. This is a phase of intimacy, or mystical marriage.

The Fifth Stage: This is passionate and illicit and is outside the bounds of normal social structures. This type of love was entered to emphasize the transcendent nature of this kind of devotion, which goes completely beyond the usual categories and forms of social conduct and conditioning.

Still farther east, the Confucian schools of China describe (in detail) the nature and rules of conduct for five main types of social relationships.

A relation of love: between father and son.

A relation of correctness and deference: between older and younger siblings.

A relation of dutiful obedience: between a ruler and his minister-advisers.

A relation of loyalty and affection: between two friends.

A relation of marriage and family: between a man and woman.

Coming full circle in our world-wide evaluation of styles of love, we return to some contemporary Western definitions. In his work, "The Styles of Loving," John Alan Lee describes six distinct patterns of feeling and behavior that his research subjects reported in their love relationships.

1. *Erotic lovers* — These types are usually taken with one another immediately. They go to bed soon after meeting a prospective partner and seek physical perfection in the experience. Erotic lovers are primarily attracted by physical beauty, with personal and intellectual qualities of secondary importance. As soon as a suitable or willing partner is found, there is an acute desire for intimacy. This type tends to be self-assured, confident, and willing to pursue ideals through many shallow relationships. Generally speaking, they are not needy, possessive, or afraid to be alone.

2. *Ludic lovers* — These are usually playful types to whom sex and love are recreational pursuits, much like athletic events. They tend to remain emotionally detached and prefer their partners not to be involved deeply with them. This type dates several people at the same time. They take care not to see anyone too often since this might ultimately limit their potential. This is the proverbial "playboy" mentality.

3. *Storgic lovers*—This is an earthier type in whom love develops slowly, quietly, and without great passion. This is the friendly, almost Platonic love that grows between people who live or work in close contact with one another. Consummation of the relationship is postponed until it is clear that marriage, home, and

children are the goals of the union. They are contrasted with the intensity of *Eros* and the playfulness of *Ludus*.

4. *Manic lovers* — This type experiences the swells and depths of the ocean of love. They tend to be consumed by thoughts of their beloved, experiencing incredible highs when things go well, and then sinking to the depths of despair if the partner seems not to respond as desired. These people live on an emotional roller coaster, full of passion, jealousy, and possessiveness. They have no control over their emotions and are "possessed" by love. They are more like erotic lovers but are less stable and independent. This is the most common type of lover.

5. *Pragmatic lovers* — This type is concerned with practicalities and lets the head rule the heart. They generally choose each other on the basis of compatibility. Common interests, backgrounds, and personalities are the important things. Intense feelings of love and devotion can develop with time, but the primary consideration is a practical match. Most marriages are based on this form of attachment.

6. *Agape lovers* —This type of lover seeks to be selfless and altruistic, surrendering personal desires to a higher ideal. This type expresses total compassion, altruism, and nondemandingness in the lover. This is the rarest form of lover; love ceases to be an addictive narcotic and a real relationship begins between two souls.

Note of Caution: *Although there are no reported poisonings from the use of muira-puama, care should be taken to determine whether there might be an allergic reaction to the resins. An allergic study can be done by scratching the skin with a sterilized pin and a sample of muira-puama. The scratches should be one-half inch long and should not draw blood. If the scratch creates* *an undesired irritation within sixty minutes, you are most likely to have an undesirable reaction to the herb.*

There are a number of other botanicals in the Olacaceae family that are commercially important. For example, the seed oil from *Ximenia americana* (West Africa) is placed in decayed teeth prior to extraction in order to facilitate removal.

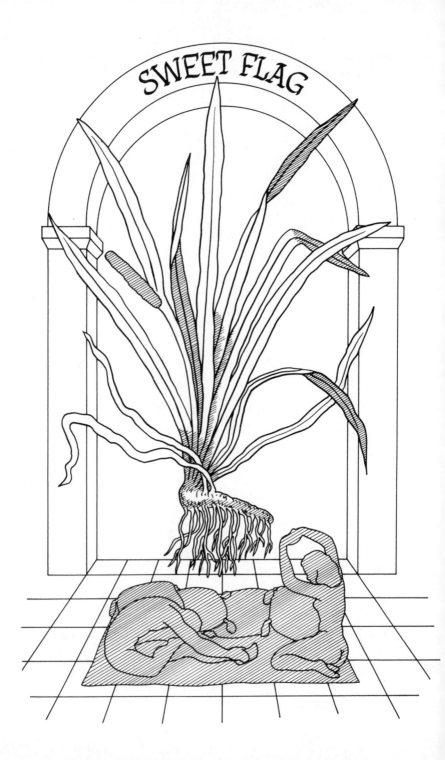

Sweet Flag

Family: Araceae (Arum).

Botanical Name: *Acorus calamus.*

Synonyms: Calamus, sweet sedge, rat root, sweet myrtle, beewort, bachh (Hindu), racha (Vedic), shih-ch'ang pu (Chinese).

Geographical Location: Europe, Asia, China, and North America; from Nova Scotia to Minnesota; southward to Florida and Texas.

Habitat: Marshes, borders of streams and ponds. Commonly seen among cattails and other species of flag.

Botanical Description: A perennial herb somewhat resembling the iris with a horizontal, creeping root stock. It may grow to be five feet long. It can be distinguished from real iris by the peculiar crimped edges of its leaves and their aromatic odor when bruised. The leaves are sword-like and grow from two to six feet high. A ridged flower stalk similar to the iris appears from the base of the outer leaves and bears

81

cylindrical blunt spike or spadix covered by minute greenish-yellow flowers.

History: Calamus has been used for over 2,000 years by the Chinese, the Moso sorcerers of Yunnan, and in the Ayurvedic systems of medicine as a remedy for bronchitis, asthma, and fevers. In China the root is ingested to relieve constipation and swelling.

The roots of this plant were also widely used by the American Indians of Canada and the United States as a medicine. A decoction of the root was drunk, the fresh root was chewed, or the root was powdered and smoked. The use of calamus in North America was analogous to the use of coca leaves *(Erthroxylon coca)* in South America. Both plants were used to combat fatigue, ward off hunger, and increase stamina.

The Cree Indians of Alberta would chew a piece of the root one to two inches in length to overcome fatigue; a ten-inch length of root was chewed to produce hallucinations and related states of consciousness. Walt Whitman wrote forty-five ballads under the title "Calamus" in his *Leaves of Grass*.

Sweet flag was also one of the constituents of an ointment that Moses was commanded to rub on his body when approaching the tabernacle:

"Moreover the Lord spoke to Moses, saying 'Take thou also unto thee the chief spice, of flowing myrrh five hundred shekels, and of sweet cinnamon half so much, even two hundred and fifty, and of sweet calamus two hundred and fifty, and of cassia five hundred, after the shekel of the sanctuary, and of olive oil a kin. And thou shall make it a holy anointing oil, an essence compounded after the art of the perfumer; it shall be a holy anointing oil.'"

EXODUS 30:22-25

Chemistry: The essential oil of sweet flag contains the psychoactive substance asarone and beta-asarone.

These are the non-amine precursors to TMA-2, a phenethylamine having ten times the potency of mescaline.

Another possible source of asorone is the wild carrot of Central Asia *(Caucus carota)*. Asarone is converted to TMA-2 in the body by aminezation, which occurs shortly after ingestion.

Approximately 1.5 to 4.5 percent of sweet flag is a bitter volatile oil. Asarone and beta-asarone make up 70 to 80 percent of this oil, the rest being eugenol, pinene, camphene, and caryophyllene.

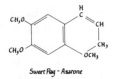

Sweet Flag - Asarone

Primary Effects: A *stimulant* when a dried root 2 inches long and the thickness of a pencil is eaten; a *hallucinogen* when over 10 inches is eaten.

Preparation: The root tastes much like ginger when dry, so that is the most common way to consume it. Your tongue will become numb for a period of four to ten minutes after eating it. A common tonic recipe is to boil 1 ounce of sweet flag root in 1 pint of water. Drink daily before meals.

The asarone is more easily converted to TMA-2 on an empty stomach. Roots deteriorate with age. They should not be used after they are two years old. The asarone has, by that time, altered itself and become useless.

Ritual Use: Throughout history and diverse cultures, there is a common belief that in order to live a prosperous and healthy life, we must tithe at least 10 percent of our life toward some form of *breath control.* Even such institutions as the American Medical Association recommend some form of aerobic exercise as necessary for a healthy lung and cardio-vascular system. Some of us do it by jogging or swimming, while others may practice Tai Chi.

Pranayama is not a new concept. It begins for each of us with the slap that causes the newborn child to take its first breath of air. The regularization of the breathing is a primary requirement and first stage of Tantric yoga. Pranayama helps to fix the attention and develops all the sense faculties, including perception, audition, touch, taste, and smell. The goal is to unite the breath power with the thought force, holding attention at the third eye.

According to yogic doctrine, pranayama, or deep rhythmic breathing, supplies us with more of the vital life forces. The basic practice of pranayama recommends holding the breath between inhalation and exhalation, going through four phases in each cycle. These minor suspensions of the breath help develop concentration. To experience the benefits of pranayama, experiment with the following exercise.

1 Sit in one of the basic yoga postures or in a straight- backed chair with feet flat on the floor, hands resting on the knees. Practice in the morning or evening on an empty stomach. Close the right nostril with the thumb of the right hand and breathe out slowly and completely through the left nostril while you count twenty seconds. Breathe in through the same nostril for ten seconds. Pause for a moment, change hands, and repeat with the other nostril. This eight-fold cycle constitutes one cycle of pranayama. Begin with five to ten cycles in the morning or evening, and gradually increase to twenty.

2. When this is quite easy, increase the periods to thirty and fifteen seconds, and increase the breath retention during the pause — but not to the point of inconvenience.

3. When this becomes fairly easy, change the exercise by breathing out for fifteen seconds, in for

fifteen seconds, and holding the breath for fifteen seconds.

4. When you can do this with perfect ease and comfort for an entire hour, practice breathing out for forty and in for twenty seconds.

5. Once this has been attained, practice breathing out for twenty, in for ten, and holding the breath for thirty seconds. When you have become efficient in this stage of pranayama, you may contemplate virtues such as love, joy, compassion, and mercy when you inhale; likewise consider the vices such as anger, lust, greed, and selfishness when you exhale. Imagine that when you inhale you absorb the virtues and when you exhale you eject the vices. Pranayama is designed to awaken the Kundalini and cause it to rise to the higher spiritual centers, or chakras. This develops concentration as well as peace of mind.

Practice pranayama in a well-ventilated room. Be careful never to strain yourself by holding the breath for an uncomfortable period of time. Increase the time gradually so you never become short of breath and gulp air unrhythmically. Various remarkable phenomena are associated with the practice of pranayama and some may occur spontaneously to you. They must be carefully analyzed and recorded for future insights into your subconscious nature. But do not dwell on these phenomena. The goal of pranayama is to develop increased concentration.

Pranayama might be used as a prelude to Tantric sexual rites. Since it is a stimulant, sweet flag will keep you alert. With an aphrodisiac more calming in nature, you might be lulled into sleep during this meditation. Sweet flag should be taken in an amount that will allow the breathing to remain controlled and regular, rather than causing it to be rapid. Remember, "your body is your temple," and sweet flag was traditionally used for approaching the tabernacle of the lord. We approach this holy ground when we concentrate our attention within.

85

Note of Caution: *Some experiments have indicated that large doses of asarone may produce tumors in rats. The amount given to produce these effects, however, is astronomical in proportion to the weight of the rat.*

Cachunde, a popular aphrodisiac in India, is taken as a lozenge. It contains sweet flag, wormwood, ambergris, and musk. It may even contain some powdered precious stones and is sold widely in India and China as a sexual stimulant, for nervous complaints, and to prolong life.

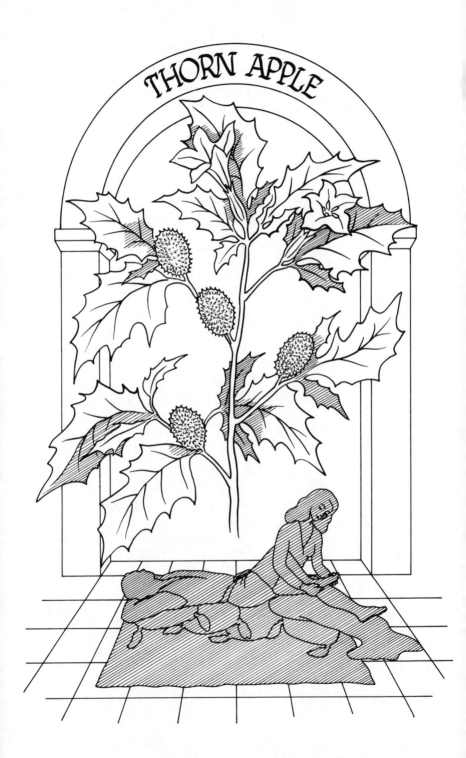

Thorn Apple

Family: Solanaceae (Potatoe).

Botanical Name: *Datura stramonium.*

Synonyms: Jimson weed, devil's apple, stinkweed, Jamestown weed, yerba del diable, angel's trumpet, Gabriel's trumpet.

Geographical Location: Native to Southwestern United States, Mexico, Central America, India, and Asia.

Habitat: Sandy soils, flatlands, open semi-dry lowland meadows and roadsides.

Botanical Description: An erect annual that grows to 4 feet in height. The leaves are 4 to 6 inches long, broad and unevenly toothed. The flowers are almost trumpet-shaped and pale blue. The plant produces large, prickly capsules filled with shiny black seeds.

History: The name *datura* originated from early Arabian names such as *datora* and *tatorah*. Early

89

Sanskrit writings refer to these drugs as *dhurstura* and *unmata*. The name "Jimson weed" comes from Jamestown, Virginia, where colonists found *datura* growing near piles of rubbish from the ships at dock.

In India, women known as "mundane ladies" (prostitutes) would use "knockout drops" *(D. metal)* for intoxicating and robbing their clients. They were probably introduced to this lifestyle by having been given the drug at an early age. It is a powerful narcotic.

Traditional techniques for witch's flying ointments used *D. stramonium* in combination with other drugs including aconite and deadly nightshade (see Mandrake chapter). The ointment was rubbed over the entire body and was absorbed through the skin and mucous membranes. This produced vivid hallucinations and experiences reported as flying on broomsticks to the Sabbath. This illusion of flying is a classic example of astral projection, similar to that described by Carlos Casteneda in *The Teachings of Don Juan,* in which the agent known as "the little smoke" was used.

Chemistry: The principle active component is a scopolamine (hyoscine). Other alkaloids are atropine, hyosyamine, mandragorine, and other tropanes. These are all parasympathetic depressants. Scopolamine is used today in several nonprescription sedatives and anti-tension preparations. In its hydrobromide form it is used for overcoming motion sickness.

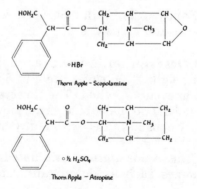

Thorn Apple – Scopolamine

Thorn Apple – Atropine

Primary Effects: Thorn apple is a parasympathetic depressant, hallucinogen, and hypnotic. Hypnotics produce low alphoid and spindal-alpha brain activity characteristic of the REM (rapid eye movement) state. It does not allow sleep to occur, although it does lower brain patterns to states in which lucid dreams do occur.

Preparation: DO NOT INGEST! Excessive amounts can be toxic. The leaves may be smoked relatively safely. *Cannabis sativa* may be added. Doses should be less than 2 grams per session, with consumption of less than one ounce each week. Even smoking may cause blacking out and severe headaches when used too often.

Ritual Use: The concept of subtle bodies created by the aspirant for experience on higher planes of consciousness is very old. Different "vehicles" are appropriate on different planes. For the physical plane, the human body is ideal. For the astral plane, the place where lucid dreams occur, an imagined *body of light* is required. This astral body of light can be thought of as a precise copy, in the finer luminous "material" of that rarified sphere, of the physical body. This light body has the ability to seemingly separate itself from the flesh and blood body, and "fly into the sky" with none of the limitations of a mortal frame.

The astral body contains the fully functioning consciousness of the aspirant. Its existence persists after physical death, and it is in this body that those who recall near-death experiences of the "other side" were functioning. The Egyptians called it the *Ka*. Magically, this astral body is built in the imagination through the process of pranayama, the control of breath (see *Sweet Flag* ritual). However, original concepts of a starry body may be traced to classical Greek philosophy, so the idea is not exclusively Oriental in origin.

There are several methods for "getting into the astral body." One technique uses a form of active *imagination* in which you develop a body of light until

91

it becomes as real to you as your physical body. The relationship between the two must become exceedingly intimate. Occult tradition asserts that these bodies are joined by a silver cord, which functions like an umbilicus. It is recommended, however, that you maintain careful differentiation between experiences in the physical and astral bodies. Astral journeys are best undertaken within a ritual format so that the results may be guided.

The first step, then, is to move the astral body outside your own physical body. You should begin by imagining a shape resembling yourself standing in front of you. Try to imagine how your physical body would look if you were standing in this place. This is tricky since you would not see the image you see in a mirror, but its reverse! Then attempt to transfer your consciousness to the body of light. Your own body should have its eyes shut. Use the eyes of the body of light to describe the objects in the room behind you.

As soon as you begin to feel more or less at home in this finer body, let it rise in the air. A good visualization is that of rising up in an elevator that is increasing in speed. A brief feeling of fear, much like the "pit of the stomach" falling sensation, will often accompany this sensation. Keep your attention on feeling that sense of rising while attempting to look about you as you rise. If possible, look at the landscape about you. The images will have a quality of their own. They are not like material things, or mental ones, but seem to have a quality between the two.

Now, however unsuccessful your attempts at getting out of the body may apparently have been, it is most important to use every effort to bring it back properly. Make the body of light coincide in space with the physical body, and then recover the unity of consciousness. If you fail to do this properly you may find yourself in psychological trouble. Any proper magical operation returns your consciousness to the point of origin (normal waking consciousness) through an *active* effort.

When in your body of light, attempt to look at your astral hands. This ability to visualize these parts of your body give you "control" of your flight, or movement within this body. By *visualizing* a merging of the two bodies (astral and physical) when completing a journey, you have a "switch" to turn your consciousness *on* and *off* during these visualization exercises. As you become more proficient at entering and leaving your body of light, you will gain a broader spectrum of awareness.

Note of Caution: *All the* daturas *can be detrimental to the heart because of the tropane alkaloids. A tolerance is built up in the parasympathetic nervous system with their continued use, thus requiring more of the plant to achieve the same "effects." This is not true with their effects on the heart, and severe damage may occur. This is why this and related tropanes should never be ingested. They are extremely toxic.*

Other tropane-containing herbs that may be used similarly are:

a) Belladonna *(Atropa belladonna),* also known as deadly nightshade. It was originally used to dilate pupils as a sign of attractiveness, hence its name belladonna.

b) Henbane *(Hysocyamus niger),* also known as devil's eye. Traditional use was as an ingredient in a flying ointment used for ritual.

c) Mandrake *(Mandragora officinarum),* also known as may apple. Believed to be magical because of the root structure's resemblance to the shape of a man.

d) Monkshood *(Aconitum napellus),* also known as wolf's bane or aconite. Traditionally considered as the most important of the solancaceae group, it was used to fight the vampire.

e) Mint Bidis (non-tobacco cigarettes from India), with the ingredients spearmint, gigantic swallow wort, thorn apple, holy basil, marjoram, sour orange, and papaval. Mint Bidis contain 65mg of scopolamine and 16 mg of atropine per cigarette.

All of the above can be made into extracts with ethyl alcohol. A smoke is then prepared by dipping a cigarette or herbal into the extract and letting it dry.

93

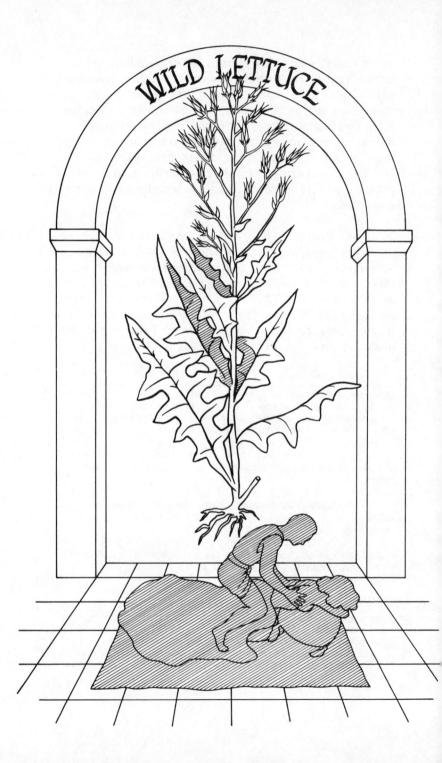

Wild Lettuce

Family: Compositae (Sunflower).

Botanical Name: *Lactuca virosa.*

Synonyms: Lettuce opium, lopium, compass plant.

Geographical Location: Southern and Central Europe and most of North America

Habitat: Loose, rich, well-drained fields.

Botanical Description: The herb is a biennial with a leafy, round stem that grows from 2 to 7 feet in height. The stem is erect and smooth, pale green, and sometimes spotted with purple. The lower leaves are large and numerous, growing to 18 inches. The upper stem leaves are small, scanty, and grow alternately. They clasp the stem with two small lobes. The heads are short stalked, with numerous pale, yellow flowers. The fruit is a rough, black oval with a broad wing along the edge that narrows to a long, white beak holding silvery tufts of hair.

History: Lettuce opium was often used by North American Indians who smoked the dried resin or sap obtained from the plant. They cut the flower heads off, gathered the sap that drained, and then let it air dry. This process was repeated over a two-week period by cutting just a little bit off the top each time.

Chemistry: Contains a milky juice known as lactucarine or lettuce opium. This compound is made up of 0.2 percent lactucin (similar in structure to opium), 50 percent lactucerol (taraxasterol), and lactucic acid, caoutchouc, a volatile oil, and mannite. Some references also report the presence of hyoscyamine, but this is not well documented. There also appears to be a high concentration of nitrates.

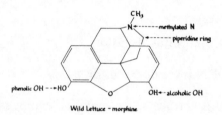

Wild Lettuce – morphine

Primary Effects: Mild narcotic and analgesic. Sedative that induces low alphoid activity rather than deep sleep. Most dream states occur in REM (rapid eye movement) sleep, a state characterized by low alphoid activity.

Preparation: The easiest method is to dry the leaves and roots and smoke them in a large pipe. A commercial preparation heats (but does not boil) the leaf in water for at least eight hours. The liquid is then removed as lactucarine is water soluble. A heat lamp is then placed over the bowl of liquid and a fan is used to drive the water out of the extraction. The result will be a blackish gum that can be smoked best with a waterpipe and hot torch.

96

The gum should be rolled in small balls and sealed in plastic to prevent drying out. The hotter the flame, the better the high. A general amount for each person is approximately 1 ounce of wild lettuce leaf, or about 1/2 to 1 gram of the extract.

Ritual Use: There is only one creative energy — *logos* — which manifests itself from its lower form, sexual energy, to the supreme spiritual or divine power. This is the true purpose of man: to raise his consciousness ever higher, to ever more spiritual levels. In order to reach the highest goal, you can accelerate the stimulation and activation of your nerve and brain centers.

The secret is already built into the body but lies in a latent condition. It is a living fire, known in Eastern philosophy as Kundalini. This living fire is expressed through your own sexual energy but can be sublimated for spiritual purposes. This energy is the link between mind and matter.

The secret of sexual energy is not only that it is capable of creating new life through the act of genera-tion, but that it has another function of vastly greater importance to man — to lead his conscious awareness step-by-step up the discrete levels of consciousness to God realization.

Creative energy alone can help man to increase the resilience of his higher nerve and brain centers and actualize the potential resting in a latent condition. These discrete stages in the ascent of consciousness from the base of the spine to the crown are given different names in different cultures. The Hindus recognize seven chakras, or centers, which could be seen as analogies of the seven rungs of the "Jacob's ladder" of consciousness. The Western magic systems orient themselves around the circuit of the tree of life, whose spheres of the middle pillar represent the four worlds, or four levels of consciousness.

Since wild lettuce promotes a languid dream state, it might be used for a magical meditation known as "rising on the planes." In this operation, the aspirant

97

visualizes himself as progressively ascending from one state of consciousness to the next higher state, moving from identification with the physical, to emotional, intellectual, and spiritual levels. This might be done during the sex act, even, beginning in a normal state and progressing to a more exalted viewpoint.

1. At the lowest rung of the ladder, man is a largely unconscious creature driven by his instincts and fate. At this level we function much like animals in an indiscriminate urge for sexual release.

2. When we awaken to the first glimmerings of consciousness, our powers of discrimination are a-wakened and we search for a partner who is physically suited to ourselves. Once such a partner is found, we seek to merge our physical needs, desires, and goals in a common direction.

3. Awakening to the astral aspects of sex enhances our emotional lives. This motivates the quest for a partner who is emotionally compatible so we may nurture and be nurtured by one another. This level of awareness awakens the bonding instinct and creates an urge to build a family unit.

4. Consciousness at the causal level of under-standing moves us to seek a mate with a compatible philosophy of life and a similar level of intelligence, as well as physical and emotional compatibility. This is a love match that has much going for it in terms of longevity.

5. This is the stage of self-realization, self-control, or mastery of one's destiny. At this stage we seek not only physical, emotional, and intellectual compatibil-ity but are also motivated to find someone who seems to embody our own internal contrasexual complement, the anima or animus. This urge comes from deep within and is in harmony with the divine laws of conscience.

People at the emotional stage confuse this with the concept of one's soul mate and may thereby be led into illusory relationships and suffer disappointment.

6. This stage represents the spiritual unity of mystical marriage, which is an internal union with one's own higher self. The experience yields a feeling of unity with the whole world and comes from the first fruits of mystical practice. We might get this same oceanic feeling during Tantric rites, which sublimate our creative energy into goals higher than that of simple release.

7. The crown of creation is experienced as a feeling of universal consciousness, also known as God realization. With this mystical union comes the supreme fulfillment of all religious meditation practices. Those who have actualized this state of consciousness are known as masters and have realized their true being and become one with God.

Note of Caution: *Homeopathic medicine recommends that anyone who suffers from any form of stomach disorder, especially ulcers, should not ingest any form of lettuce. This is due to the fact that all lettuces, including garden varieties, contain this lettuce opium product that will coat the stomach wall and inhibit the digestion process.*

A decoction of the leaf serves as an excellent face wash.

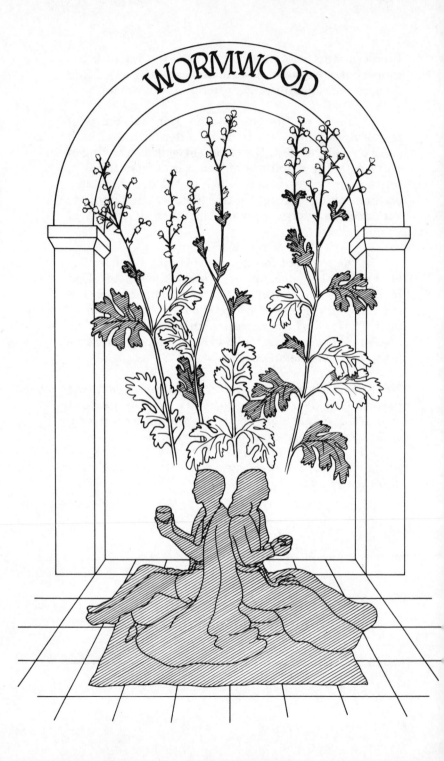

Wormwood

Family: Compositae (Sunflower or Aster).

Botanical Name: *Artemisia absinthium.*

Synonyms: Absinthe, green ginger, "the devil's liquor," "green muse."

Geographical Location: In most parts of the world, from the United States to Siberia.

Habitat: Roadsides, waste areas, and near the sea.

Botanical Description: A silky, perennial plant supported by a woody root stock producing many bushy stems that grow from 2 to 4 feet in height. The stems are whitish and are closely covered with fine, silk hairs. The leaves are also hairy and are shaped with many blunt lobs of an irregular greenish-yellow color that are arranged on an erect, leafy flower stem. The leaves and flowers have a very bitter taste and a characteristic odor.

History: The genus is named *Artemisia* from Artemis, the Greek name for Diana, goddess of the moon. The plant was of some importance among Mexicans, who celebrated their great festival of the goddess of salt by a ceremonial dance of women who wore garlands of wormwood on their heads.

An old love charm recommends that on St. Luke's Day one should cut marigold flowers, sprigs of marjoram, thyme, and a little wormwood. These are dried before a fire and rubbed to a powder. They are then simmered over a slow fire in a small quantity of honey (virgin) and vinegar. You should then anoint yourself with this mixture when going to bed, saying the following:

"St. Luke, St. Luke, be kind to me,
In dreams let me my true-love see."

Chemistry: Absinthine (a dimeric guaranolide), the principal agent, and anabsinthin, and thujone $(C_{10}H_{16}O)$. Absinthine is listed as a narcotic analgesic in the same group as codeine and dextromethorphan hydrobromide (Romilar).

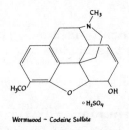

Wormwood – Codeine Sulfate

Absinthe is a green-colored liquor flavored with oil of wormwood, anise *(Pimpinella anisum),* marjoram *(Origanum majorana),* elecampane *(Inula helenium),* and several other herbs. This concoction has an almost instaneous aphrodisiac effect on both men and women, also acting much like a narcotic.

The maximum non-lethal dose (orally) of thujone is 75 mg per kg of body weight. It is not as toxic as reported, with the intake of thujone in one ounce of

102

traditional absinthe (drunk by a 150 pound person) being 50 times less than the dosage required to cause a minimum toxic reaction. Most now consider the most harmful ingredient in absinthe not to be wormwood or thujone, but the drinking alcohol, ethanol.

Primary Effects: Narcotic-analgesic, affecting the cerebral cortex of the brain. It depressed the central medullary part of the brain, the area concerned with pain and anxiety.

Preparation: The herb is either smoked or prepared as a liqueur. Absinthine can be extracted with alcohol and water. Thujone is definitely toxic and is now classified by our government as a poison. Before the United States approves any liquor formula, it must be *almost* 100 percent thujone free. Why *almost* free? Because vermouth also contains thujone. When wormwood is used in vermouth and is extracted, it is a wine and of low proof. A minimum percentage of thujone is present. However, when wormwood is macerated for forty-eight hours or longer in neutral spirits and is then redistilled, the result is a high percentage of thujone. Thujone is not soluble in low proof; the higher the proof, the higher the concentration of thujone.

It is these minute percentages of thujone in vermouth that give the ubiquitous martini its aphrodisiac reputation. Anisette or Pernod has often been substituted for absinthe in the marketplace. Pernod does not inebriate a person as quickly as absinthe, being 40 to 50 percent alcohol, but it tastes much the same. Except for the anise used to replace the banned oil of wormwood, it contains all the same ingredients, yet the essential thujone is conspicuously absent.

Ritual Use: Absinthe, an alcoholic decoction of various herbs, was popular among artists, writers, and poets of *fin de siecle* Paris during the Impressionist movement. It gained quite a reputation as an aphrodisiac as well as a source of artistic inspiration.

Prior to this period, painting was rigidly controlled by the aesthetic criteria of the classical academy style and largely imitated the old masters of the Renaissance who took their inspiration from classical Greece. The Impressionists broke with this style by trying to capture the essence of a scene through the play of light and color. Absinthe was instrumental in helping to create this revisioning of artistic style.

Degas was one who use and "knew" his absinthe. Ten years before he painted *absintheurs,* Edouard Manet, then leader of the Impressionist movement, cautioned him to stop "painting classical Greek bullshit and concentrate on rendering just what the eye sees."

Impressionism was the first artistic movement organized entirely in cafes. Therefore, Impressionism and absinthe became synonymous. Perceptions irrigated by great quantities of absinthe transposed the world into a series of points, dots, smudges, washes, and smears. Rimbaud claimed that by deliberate intoxication, the conscious mind would open to the ineffable. This point is debatable, but the narcotic properties certainly produced a vivid imagery state while the removal of pain and anxiety might have lent the driven artist a taste of euphoria. By drinking absinthe, it was alleged that the poet could achieve a fusion of all the senses, a perfect synesthesia in which to dream.

When the poet dreams of his true love, it generally means his muse, or his art, and he is a very devout lover. By tradition, the time between four and six o'clock in the evening was designated the "hour of the aperitif," and the proper aperitif to drink was, of course, absinthe. The favorite vantage points for "being seen" and people watching were along the sidewalks under awnings.

A waiter would appear when you called "Garcon! Garcon!" He would squeeze through the crowd and place an empty tumbler on the table in front of you. Inside was a smaller jigger containing an ounce of dark, green absinthe. It was 136 proof and considered much too strong to drink unless diluted.

The ritual continued as the waiter then dripped water into the emerald elixer until it overflowed from the one container into the other. This changed the color from luminous green to a milky opalescence. The ceremony continued until the jigger held nothing but clear water. This meant that the contents of the tumbler would be five parts water to one part absinthe. This was considered the proper aperitif for all occasions.

Because of the modern restrictions on the use of absinthe and wormwood products, our easiest access to the state of consciousness embodied in Impressionism lies through appreciation of the art of this period. Maybe you and your loved one can share a martini or two and stroll through an exhibition of these beautiful works. Perhaps a trip to Paris could be an aphrodisiac in itself!

Note of Caution: *Excessive long-term use of absinthe may be habit-forming and debilitating. Ingestion of the thujone or wormwood volatile oils as a tincture may cause gastro-intestinal disturbances and convulsions due to the thujone.*

Thujone is still present today in vermouth (from the German *Wermut,* which means wormwood). It is legally permissible in quantities of 10 ppm. There are 60 ppm of thujone in absinthe. (Thujone is also present in sage.)

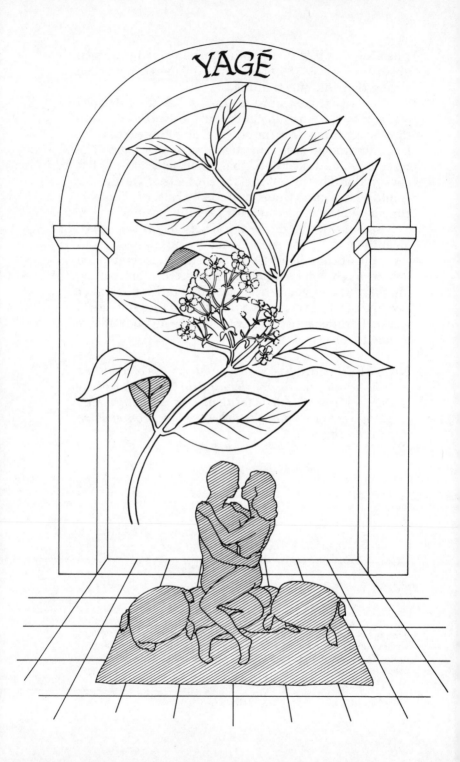

A psychic energizer
and sex stimulant

Yage'

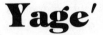

Family: Malpighiaceae.

Botanical Name: *Banisteriopsis caapi* M.

Synonyms: Ayahuasca, cappi, natem pinde.

Geographical Location: The Amazon basin of Brazil, along the Pacific coast of Colombia, throughout Ecuador, and in parts of Peru.

Habitat: Rain forests and jungles.

Botanical Description: An extensive vine hanging from jungle trees. The bark is somewhat raised and textured. The leaves are egg-shaped and are lanced at the ends; they are about 3.5 inches long and 2 inches wide. The flowers are carmine-pink in axillary panicles. The petals fall quickly and the fruit is a reddish- brown winged seed.

History: The Indian tribes of the South American Orinoco and Amazon Basin regions use yage' in their ceremonials. They believe that the intoxication it produces marks a "return to earth," a return to the beginning of things. The experience is a ceremonial fortification of the religious concepts of the Indians.

The Tukanoans of Colombia administer the drug to adolescent boys to fortify them against the pain and shock of their ritual entry into the state of manhood. The use of *ayahuasca* by these same tribes sometimes involved flagellation and may be heavy in sexual content. In Brazil and Peru, yage′ becomes a part of the deeply religious ceremonies that are linked to early tribal legends and mythology. Peruvian witch doctors use the plant to diagnose and treat diseases. This narcotic drink was widely employed in northern South America for prophecy, divination, and as a magical hallucinogen.

A number of studies have confused ayahuasca, caapi, and yage′as substances other than *Banisteriopsis caapi*. These include *Haemadictyon amazonicum* and *Datura suaveolens*. Further studies, however, indicate that these different plants were added to *B. caapi* or *B. inebrians* to enhance the total effect of the drug. B. rusbyana leaves contain N,N-dimethyltriptamine in relatively high concentrations. This mixture was known as *oco-yage*′ The natives added these leaves to "heighten and lengthen" the visual experiences.

The natives of Rio Napo commonly consumed a mixed extract of the B. *caapi* and *Prestonia amazonica (Haemadictyon amazonicum)* in the belief that the latter suppressed the more unpleasant hallucinations associated with the pure *B. caapi* extracts. This was a more soothing concoction since the MAO-inhibitors enhance the effects of the calming tryptamines.

Chemistry: Yage′contains the unusual psychoactive beta- carbolines harmine, harmaline, and d-tetrahydroharmine. In addition to acting upon the central nervous system, harmine and the related harmaline and harmalol have produced sexual responses in rats under laboratory conditions when given 5 mg of harmine.

Small doses of harmine (25 to 75 mg subcutaneously) produce euphoria in man. Harmine is effective in doses of 500 to 700 mg, with harmaline doses less than half this amount. The harmal alkaloids are most effective if used in combination rather than singly.

All of the harmal alkaloids act upon the central nervous system. One of them, 6-methoxytetrahydro-harmane, is found in the pineal gland in human and other animals. There is some belief that this chemical is somewhat more abundant in the pineal (so-called "third eye") gland of highly advanced yogis and other mediators. Production of this substance is said to increase with spiritual development.

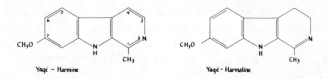

Yagé – Harmine   Yagé – Harmaline

Primary Effects: Most experience nausea, and some vomit before the effects begin to show. Effects begin about one hour after ingestion and persist for up to eight hours. The kaleidoscopic phenomena common with other indolic alkaloids such as LSD and psilocybin do not seem to occur. Perception of the environment remains essentially unchanged. However, images often appear superimposed on background surfaces, and imaginary scenes are seen simultaneously. Closed-eye imagery is usually vivid and brightly colored. Long, dreamlike sequences are also common. Time sense and music perception are not noticeably altered. Harmala alkaloids are short-term MAO inhibitors.

Small amounts of the drug act as a psychic energizer and sex stimulant. Larger doses can produce brilliant hallucinations, illusions of size changes in objects, and unusually keen night vision. Excessive amounts were known to produce nightmare visions and a psychotic state.

Preparation: The stem is pounded in a mortar, usually with other local psychoactive materials (mostly

109

solanaceous plants). These are then boiled in a small amount of water for 8 hours, strained, and reduced to 1/10 the original volume. Four-ounce cups of this liquid can be taken, but beginners should start with only one ounce. The amount of total harmal alkaloid in a 4-ounce cup is approximately 500 mg.

The harmal alkaloids are very poorly absorbed through the stomach and intestines. Twenty-five to 100 mg of harmine hydrochloride can be taken as a snuff to produce almost immediate results. Unfortunately, the drug produces a terrible burning of the nostrils and throat, which leaves one for several days with all of the nose and throat symptoms of a cold. The best way to use the pure alkaloid is to place the same amount (25 to 100 mg) of the substance under the tongue and between the gums and the lips where it is readily absorbed.

Ritual Use: Witnesses of the various Indian yage' ceremonies report great *empathy* among the celebrants. In fact, they all frequently see the same visions simultaneously. Many persons have noted what seems to be an increase in ESP ability while under the influence of the drug. This is one reason the original isolated alkaloid was first called *telepathine* or *banisterine,* then later called harmaline.

Empathic states of consciousness are those in which there is intellectual or emotional identification with another. It is a subjective point of resonance between two or more persons. Men and women are always communicating one way or another; every one of their words, gestures, actions, intonations, and sounds says something to the other party. Whether or not it is saying what he or she thinks is being communicated is quite another matter.

There is no guaranteed way to avoid misunderstandings with a mate. But one thing is certain: coaxing, cajoling, dropping "cute" hints, manipulation, and beating around the bush are all barriers to clear communication. When messages are hidden, when you don't quite say what you mean but subtly allude to it, you are leaving yourself open to misinterpretation. Misinterpretations build, and entrenched patterns of indirectness develop.

One of the major casualties of our busy, preoccupied lives has been empathy. The most refined form of feeling-oriented communication, empathy is an effort to understand each other's beliefs, practices, feelings, and perspective without necessarily sharing or agreeing with them. It is as if an individual were silently asking, "How does that other person see it? How does that other person feel? How would I feel if what I am saying to her were said to me?"

While empathy does not require agreement with the other's view, it does preclude the demand, "You must think, feel, and act like me." There are two techniques to remember in developing empathy:

1. Listening and attempting to understand the other person's point of view rather than busily preparing your own rebuttal;

2. Communicating this understanding to the speaker.

Whenever differences occur, whether between spouses, business partners, or nations, they are resolved in only one of three ways: attempted domination by one party (result: hostility, war); mutual or unilateral withdrawal (result: divorce, isolation); mutual compromise (result: something for everybody).

If individuals are seeking a relationship with each other more satisfying than aggression and divorce, mutual exchange and compromise clearly offer the greatest promise. Here are some rules for renegotiating and compromising moderately abrasive differences before they become severe.

1. If you are both busy going your separate ways and have many other time commitments, set aside a time for a formal meeting specifically for the compromise-exchange discussion. If one partner keeps postponing the meeting, it may be a way of silently

protesting or avoiding confrontation. Discuss this issue.

2. Each participant must state very specifically, in positive terms, exactly what he or she needs, desires, and expects. Be sure to avoid vague generalities which could later be misinterpreted.

3. Begin by saying what you want, not what you don't, won't, or can't tolerate. Take equal responsibility for the condition of the relationship and avoid using the exchange ritual as a forum for condemning the behavior of the other. Reinforce positive behavior through encouragement, and stick to a "no- fault" rule, which does not pass-the-buck by putting the blame on one partner only. There are two sides to every story, and this session seeks to consider and define those differences.

4. Do not attempt to manipulate the other's feelings; they probably can't help how they feel about things. However, behavior that is annoying or counter-productive can be negotiated if it does not compromise a person's integrity. Compromise within the situation rather than by bartering emotions. Emotional blackmail usually boomerangs anyway.

5. Remain cool and be patient! No one is likely to give up their stubborn position without a fight. Stick to the current topic; don't tangent into past arguments. Take the time to come to an exchange of perspectives and work out a compromise. Mutual agreement may come only after several discussions.

Sharing a cup of yage' one hour before these planned discussions can make the empathic sharing more real and productive. When using these harmala alkaloids, one is able to experience the inter-individual communication and perception with a lover. It is as if the collective unconscious of the two becomes an immediate reality. This empathy was a primary reason for the use of yage' in diverse Indian ceremonies conducted for spiritual reasons. In their primitive environment, survival often depended upon the good will and understanding of another. The same might be said of our modern, urban life-styles.

Characteristically, the drug intensifies the ability to telepathize and enhances extrasensory perception beyond the usual conscious levels. Such simultaneous vision perceptions move one toward those desired empathetic states of consciousness that lead to inter-personal harmony.

Note of Caution: *Harmala alkaloids are mild MAO inhibitors. (See Yohimbe, Note of Caution).*

There are several other harmine-containing plants:

1. Syrian rue *(Peganum harmala)* is found through-out the Mediterranean area and in parts of the Middle East, Central Asia, and North Africa. Large patches can also be found now in parts of Texas and the American Southwest. Turkish red dye, the pigment used in Turkish and Persian carpets, is made from the seeds. (In Egypt the oil extract from the seed is sold as an aphrodisiac under the name *Zit-el-Harmel.)*

2. Wild rue or Syrian bean-caper (Zygophyllum fabago) can be found in deserts of the western coast of the United States. Native to the Old World, they were introduced and established in such places as Ephrata, Washington, and Minidoka, Idaho.

3. Passion flower *(Passiflora incarnata)* grows in temperate areas throughout the world. The Catholics, when the plant was first introduced in Europe, saw it as a symbolic representation of the "passion of Christ."

All the seeds and leaves of these plants contain the beta-carboline alkaloids harmine, harmaline, and related bases. Isomer harmaline has been used for Parkinson's disease. It is a very potent MAO inhibitor.

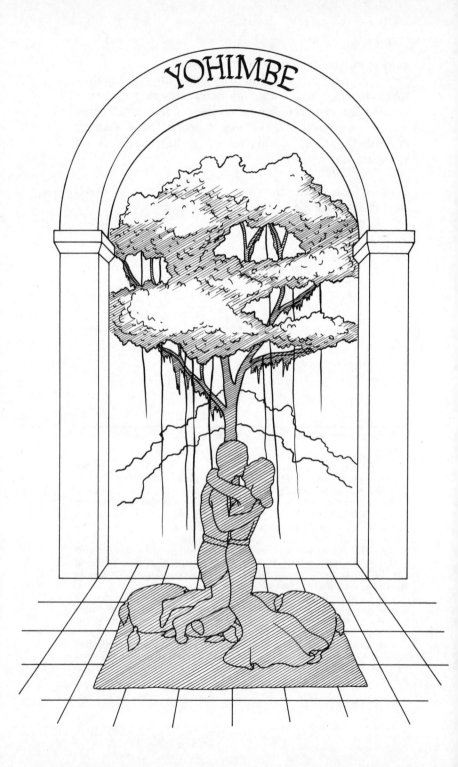

Yohimbe

Family: Rubiaceae (Madder).

Botanical Name: *Corynanthe yohimbe.*

Synonyms: Pausinystalia yohimba, yohimbehe, jo-
himbe.

Geographical Location: Tropical West Africa, especially the French Congo and the Cameroons.

Habitat: Jungle forests, low altitude.

Botanical Description: A large tree that grows from
20 to 50 feet in height. The leaves are 3 to 5 inches in
length and are oblong and oval in shape. The seeds are
winged.

History: It is traditionally used by most of the Bantu-
speaking tribes as a sacrament for pagan matrimony,
the inner shavings of the bark acting as a stimulant
and aphrodisiac. It is only used when mate rituals
occur. These orgy rituals have been known to continue
for up to ten or even fifteen days, with gradually increasing doses.

115

Chemistry: The active constituents are yohimbine, yohimbiline, and ajmaline, all indole-based alkaloids. The major alkaloid yohimbine can also appear as a hydrochloride. This makes it easily assimilated through the mucous membranes in the nose or sublingually under the tongue.

Yohimbine and yohimbiline must react with the hydrochloric acid in the digestive juices to become soluble and be assimilated into the body. Yohimbine hydrochloride is also known as quebrachine. Quebrachine can be found in the evergreen Quebracho tree that grows throughout South America. It is used primarily to reduce fever.

Yohimbe bark, strychnine, and methyl testosterone are combined in the medical preparations known as "afrodex" and "potensanforte." They are considered "limited" in their medical effectiveness.

Yohimbine is also found in *Alchornea floribunda,* an African plant that is a member of the spurge family. The root bark is usually macerated and powdered.

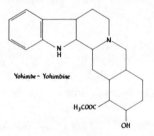

Yohimbe ~ Yohimbine

Primary Effects: Yohimbe acts both as a central nervous-system stimulant and as a mild hallucinogen. Yohimbine is a sympatho-mimetic indole-type alkaloid with cholinergic adrenergic blocking properties. It also inhibits serotonin.

The first effects are a lethargic weakness of the limbs and a vague restlessness, similar to the initial effects of LSD. Chills and warm spinal shivers may also be felt, along with slight dizziness and nausea.

116

There is a similar reaction in people who ingest such drugs as MDA (methaldyamphetamine). Then the effects produce a relaxed, somewhat inebriated mental and physical feeling accompanied by slight auditory/ visual hallucinations. Spinal ganglia are then affected, causing erection of the sex organs. These effects last from two to four hours.

Preparation: There are several techniques for preparing yohimbe. The traditional way (per person) is to bring 2 cups of water to a boil. One ounce of yohimbe is then added to the boiling water and allowed to boil for less than 4 minutes. The heat should then be turned down and the brew allowed to simmer for an additional 20 minutes. Strain the liquid and sip slowly about one hour before the effects are desired.

If you add 1,000 mg of ascorbic acid (Vitamin C), the bark tea will react to form yohimbine and yohimbiline ascorbate. These are very soluble forms of the two alkaloids. They are more efficient in this state in that they are more easily assimilated by the body and the possible nausea tends to be reduced. It is also recommended that you fast for an 18-hour period prior to ingestion.

The second technique is much more efficient. For one person, soak 1 ounce of yohimbe bark shavings in ethyl alcohol or any drinking alcohol (gin or vodka) for an 8-hour period. Strain the shavings, pour the liquid onto a flat sheet, and let the alcohol evaporate. You may use an oven at low heat (150 to 250°F) to speed evaporation. The residue, amounting to 1 to 1.5 grams, will be primarily yohimbine hydrochloride. This can be snuffed or placed under the tongue. The effects are more pronounced and the reaction occurs within 10 to 20 minutes rather than after one hour.

Ritual Use: Yohimbe is the finest sacrament that can be used for a "pagan" wedding ceremony. A complete ritual can be found in the companion text *The Magical and Ritual Use of Herbs* (Destiny Books); the Yohimbe bark is used in the sacrament. While this ceremony is not legally binding and requires a civil wedding to be legal, the mystic vows made seem decidedly more binding.

Pagan marriages are celebrated in a lovely old ceremony known as "handfasting." The sense of touch is cultivated as part of the ritual. From early youth, a child in a pagan home is taught to pet animals "with love in your hands." The creature's response is a living gauge of success, and eventually an important lesson is learned. The ability to heal, to comfort, and to love develops apace with a growing awareness that thought can be transmitted by touch.

It is, therefore, a natural nuptial rite of passage for pagans to symbolize this aspect by the clasping of hands, or handfasting. Today the handfasting union can mean anything the couple chooses to make it mean, but it is understood that the ritual itself can set in motion psychic forces that cannot be reversed. In the words of one Alexandrian High Priest: "And now, as I join your hands, I betrothe your souls."

The union becomes complete when "To find the other is to find oneself. . .", or by reunion with the immortal beloved, you discover your real self. During the handfast, mentally interlock your bodies and form a single body with your mind's eye. At first, simply extend your attention over your own body, running your awareness up and down, separating the sensations of your body from your partner's. Feel and sense your own body.

Next begin to allow your body sensing to flow into your partner's body, sensing that body as if it were part of your own. Accept the feelings and sensations of your partner's body, no matter what it feels like to you. Most important, accept that it is possible to do this.

Connect the sense of being in both bodies at once, and flow your awareness through both bodies as if they were a single form. See yourself as having one large body with four arms and two heads. Later, while in bed, repeat this exercise but with a slight modification. When you initially interlock your bodies physically, lie back, forming a single body with a head at each end. During this exercise it is important not to move once in position.

Note of Caution: *Yohimbe is a MAO inhibitor (monamine oxidase). Among the materials that may be dangerous in combination with MAO inhibitors are sedatives, tranquilizers, antihistamines, narcotics, and large quantities of alcohol. Any of these will cause hypotensive crisis (severe blood pressure drop). Amphetamines, LSD, cocaine, dairy products including aged cheese ... any of these will cause hypertensive crisis (severe blood pressure rise). It is generally recommended that* no other drug *be used in combination with or within a ten-hour period of the use of yohimbe.*

Librium or sodium amobarbitol partially block yohimbe effects. Indian snakeroot *Rauwolfice serpentina)* also contains yohimbine and indole alkaloids. Rauwolfia is not recommended as it takes a minimum of two days to several weeks for the body to metabolize reserpine. There is no control over when the effect will occur. It is quite dangerous as an MAO inhibitor.

PART II

"The first and foremost erogenous zone is in the mind."

Anatole Broyard, from a review
of a recent D'Annunzio biography

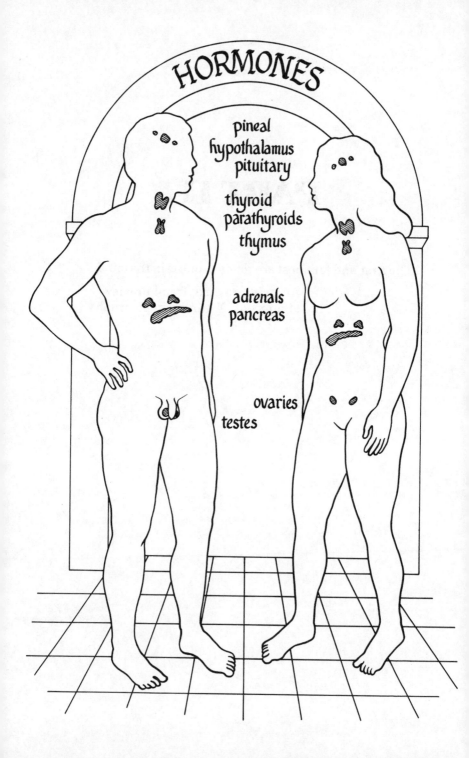

HORMONES

pineal
hypothalamus
pituitary

thyroid
parathyroids
thymus

adrenals
pancreas

ovaries
testes

Hormones

The word *hormone* was first used in 1904 by the English physiologist Dr. Ernest Starling. It was derived from a Greek word meaning "to excite" or "to set in motion." Dr. Starling defined the hormone as a chemical compound formed by certain body structures, usually from the endocrine glands. It was believed to travel through the body via the blood, influencing the growth, development, and function of other parts of the body. This definition is still used today. For a better perspective, we should first look at the brain.

The Brain

The human brain is a three-pound lump of pinkish-gray tissue. In some areas of the brain, the neurons are packed as densely as 2.4 million cells per cubic millimeter. This body of neurons comprises the brain's gray matter, and their long nerve fibers, covered with fatty, pale insulation, make up the white matter.

Neurons cannot repair themselves when damaged. A neuron that has been lost due to age or injury is gone forever. We are, in essence, born with all the neurons we will ever have. Fortunately, the brain seems quite redundant in its organization. Although neurons die at the rate of about 1,000 per day, mental acuity does not decline detectably until quite late in life.

At the core of the brain is the so-called "reptilian brain." This regulates vital functions of the body, such as heartbeat, blood pressure, breathing, and digestion. It gives rise to primitive, instinctual behavior patterns and is now known as the primitive brain.

Wrapped around the primitive brain is the "limbic system." This structure enables us to behave in a motivated, goal-directed manner. The paired brain hemispheres are covered with a thin, convoluted mantle of neocortex (the most recent product of evolution). This layer of cells (only 2.5 millimeters thick) is responsible for our ability to think, to communicate with one another, and to experience subtle emotional states such as love.

What links the body to the brain? Hormones are still viewed as the culprits in a wide range of nonphysical disturbances. Although we cannot see or feel our hormones, when the changes of adolescence and monthly menstrual periods occur, we can't miss them for the importance they have in the body.

The Endocrine System

The combined weight of the endocrine glands is only two ounces. The word *endocrine* is derived from two Greek words meaning "inside separation" or "internal secretion." Other glands in the body, such as the kidneys and the sweat glands, secrete substances through specialized tubes. These glands are called *exocrine* (outside separation) *glands*.

The hormones secreted by the endocrine glands profoundly affect every aspect of human physiology, from growth to metabolism, organ functioning, sexuality, and fertility. Scattered strategically throughout the body, these thirteen endocrine glands operate under the control of what used to be called the master gland, or *pituitary*.

124

We now know that the pituitary gland plays a secondary role to a part of the brain called the *hypothalmus gland.* The hypothalmus acts as a composer for the pituitary, just as the pituitary is the conductor over the other endocrine glands. The pituitary is located in the base of the brain and secretes at least nine different known substances. The hormones of the pituitary act directly on other endocrine glands and are called *tropic* or *trophic* hormones (from the Greek word "to turn" or "to change"). For example, the hormone of the pituitary that causes changes in the production of sex hormones of the gonads is called *gonadotrophin.*

Most of these substances from the pituitary are called *releasing hormones,* chemicals with no other purpose than to notify the endocrine glands to start secreting their own individual hormones. The pituitary's own function is to regulate growth via the growth hormone *HGH.*

Also located in the brain is the *pineal gland.* It seems to be light sensitive and is responsible for our natural body cycles and the daily ebb and flow of all hormones. While the seasonal changes might affect this gland, it certainly follows that artificial lighting may seriously alter our relationship to seasonal changes and our immune system's response to those triggers.

The *thyroid gland,* set astride the windpipe, is responsible for metabolism (the conversion of food into energy). This gland can be likened to the accelerator of a car, determining how quickly or slowly a system functions. An overactive thyroid will leave us restless, excitable, and irritable, while an underactive one produces a tired, sluggish feeling.

The four *parathyroid* glands, the smallest of the endocrine glands, are each about the size of a grain of rice. Located adjacent to the thyroid, they are responsible for the proper metabolism of calcium and phosphorus.

Perched atop the kidneys are the *adrenal glands,* producing (among other things) a hormone called *epinephrine.* Known also as *adrenalin,* epinephrine is responsible for our "fight or flight" responses.

The *pancreas gland* is the most complex of the glands. While the bulk of it manufactures digestive juices, a group of cells known as the *islets of Langerhans* produces both insulin and glycogen for metabolizing carbohydrates, proteins, and fats.

The *sex glands (ovaries* in the female, *testes* in the male) are the final endocrine glands.

The Sex Hormones

The endocrine glands that produce hormones involved in sex and reproduction are the pituitary, the adrenals, and the gonads (testes and ovaries). Most of these sex hormones are of a type called *steroids.* The shape of the basic building block of all steroid molecules is hexagonal. The small groups of molecules attached to the steroid identify it and determine its effects. Not all steroids are sex hormones, however.

The steroid hormones produced by the gonads and adrenals are the primary sex hormones. They fall into three main categories—androgens, estrogens, and *progestins.* Androgens are usually thought of as the male sex hormones because they are the predominate sex hormone produced by males. The word *androgen* is derived from the Greek word for "man" or "male." All three forms appear in both men and women, however.

Androgens include such well-known substances as *testosterone* and *androsterone.* Androgens produced at puberty stimulate development of secondary sexual characteristics. They also develop and maintain the testes and the production of sperm and help produce a positive nitrogen balance that assists growth and improves muscle tone. *LHRH* (a human hormone factor) is a luteinizing hormone-releasing substance that has been found to increase production of testosterone in men. Other natural sources include sarsaparilla root *(Smilax medica).*

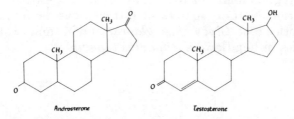

Androsterone   Testosterone

Testosterone is valuable in helping to overcome the sexual impotence of aging, the natural weakening of manly sexual vigor under the onslaught of advancing years. The value of this hormone is primarily for those middle-aged and older, where sexual potency is becoming deficient. For those undergoing the dreaded syndrome of aging, with the accompanying loss of sexual powers, an internal dose of powdered sarsaparilla root of five to fifteen grains, two to four times each day can be taken.

Estrogen and progestins are usually thought of as the female sex hormones because they are predominately found in women. *Estrogen* is derived from the Latin and Greek word for "frenzy." *Progestin* originates from the Latin words *pro* ("for") and *gest* ("gestation" or pregnancy"). High levels of these hormones are associated with behavior thought to be typical of women.

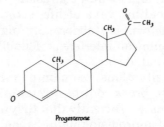

Progesterone

In women the primary source of androgens is the adrenal cortex, although ovaries can also produce

127

them. Similarly, in men, the testes produce estrogens and progestins as well as androgens. The main estrogens found in women are *estradiol, estrone,* and *estriol.* Natural sources of estrogen can be found in licorice root *(Glycyrrhiza glabra),* and in smaller quantities in hop flowers *(Humulus lupulus).*

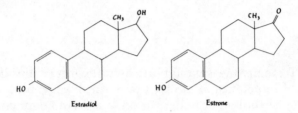

Estradiol   Estrone

Rheumatism root *(Dioscarea villosa)* contains a saponin (dioscin). The aglycone of dioscin (diosgenin) is a steroid base from which progesterone and cortisone are now manufactured. Other reputed natural sources for the female sex hormones are the saw palmetto berries *(Serenoa serrulata),* "dong kwai" *(Angelica polymorpha-Chinese),* and *bee pollen.*

Serotonin Inhibitors

Serotonin is a neurochemical of which the body produces small but necessary amounts. Overproduction can bring on unpleasant symptoms such as dizziness, exhaustion, nausea, headaches, irritability, poor judgment, and mental confusion. Because of our generally unhealthy ways of life, serotonin levels in most urban humans are abnormally high. This abundance of serotonin can interfere profoundly with normal sexual desires and abilities.

In such situations, serotonin inhibitors (substances which break down serotonin) can restore sexual functions so efficiently that they often appear to have an almost aphrodisiac quality about them. *L-dopa* (used in the treatment of Parkinson's disease) is derived from *dihydroxyphenylalanine* and is a powerful serotonin inhibitor. Although it is true that most instances of impotence, frigidity, and diminished sexual interest are psychological in origin, it should be remembered that psychological stress brings about biochemical imbalances.

Sexual awareness is the natural state of humans, but it can be subdued by stress-inducing excesses of serotonin. Sexual desire is often best rekindled not through stimulation and stimulants but by removal of the serotonin blocks that hinder our normal desire. *There is little to be gained from other aphrodisiacs and sex enhancers until serotonin levels are normalized.*

Ritual Use

Just as animals have courting rituals, so humans have instinctual courting habits. These are motivated by the endocrine system via hormones. They reflect biological as well as psychological principles. Many of these courting rituals and so-called "love signals" are a direct result of various hormones and their activity in our bodies.

Gestures alone represent more than 75 percent of our nonverbal communication and behavior. Courtship is a nonstop activity wherever men and women gather. A brief understanding of some of the rules can be of tremendous help when interacting with the opposite sex. The following ritual gestures are just a few of the rules that help to give a broader perspective of this form of communication.

1. The classic shrug of the shoulders is known as the "I give up" gesture. Both men and women unconsciously raise their shoulders when they find each other attractive. Women usually raise theirs higher than men.

2. "A coy look" is given when one is attracted to another and the head is then tilted down and to one side. This gesture is then completed by looking directly back at the person of interest.

3. Watching people's feet determines where they rate in a pecking order. This is a component of the

startle reflex and is a submissive display. If your boss pats you on your back, your feet will probably be pigeon-toed inward. As he talks to you, his feet will probably be toed out. With a man and a woman, both will often turn their toes inward. This mirroring of gestures indicates that they are comfortable with each other.

4. Smiling evolved from the "fear grimace," an expression of appeasement among primates (most often seen with monkeys). If an animal is on the weak side, its best strategy is to appease.

5. Swaying slightly as you talk has a soothing, calming effect, just as it does with babies. It seems to lessen the anxiety that accompanies courtship.

6. The qualities that women look for in men are not those that men look for in women. Men look for a woman who is physically attractive, while women look for signs of kindness and status in men. Men's clothing is part of this courtship strategy. A western-style business suit, for example, appeals to women because it signifies status. Because the jacket reaches a man's fingertips, it makes his upper body look a third again as large as it actually is. Buttoned-suit jackets with lapels make the chest look massive.

7. Women's clothing and make-up are used to compete for a man's attention. This is done to enhance youthful traits and physical attractiveness. Women's blouses, for example, have puffed sleeves, which suggest the submissive cue of lifted shoulders. This makes the woman easier to approach. Her high heels are an even more blatant courtship signal. They shift her center of gravity and force her to angle her hips to the rear, requiring a compensating forward thrust of the rib cage. All this makes her hindquarters protrude and her breasts jut out.

8. A classic stance between a man and a woman can be seen when the female is facing the male directly and he is looking out toward the distance. This indicates that the woman is more concerned with the personal relationship while the male is more concerned

with the world at large. Traditional roles of both have always emphasized that the feminine aspect was toward domestication, while the masculine aspect was toward expansion of territory.

9. A giant tilt of the head indicates that the couple is still communicating too much to be an established couple. They are more than likely also standing apart with this type of gesture, rather than holding hands. This is a way in which to determine relationships from a distance.

10. Holding hands, with fingers linked, indicates that the couple is not testing the distance between them emotionally. They have already negotiated "closeness." If they did not know each other well, they would be testing each other with such things as walking fast, trying new positions, laughing, and in some other forms of anxiety.

11. Blaring music from someone's window or automobile is a territorial signal similar to a dog spraying a tree with his scent. Other forms of this behavior can be seen along "Greek row" on most campuses. In animals, males gather at a lek, a place where they show off for the females. The females will watch their antics from the sidelines until they have enough information to pick the best male.

12. Staking out territory is often seen in bars, where the male will come to a spot at the bar, put his cigarettes on the table, or pile some money (including bills) or his keys in order to stake a claim. A man's urge to claim territory is an unconscious way of showing females his status relative to other males.

Note of Caution: *There is a relationship between noradreneline-serotonin cycles in the body. For as excited (or high) as one gets, there must be a balance of becoming depressed (or low) in order for the body to achieve a balance (or homeostasis). This cycle is usually two to three days in length and explains why most true meditators attempt to maintain a neutral emotional relationship with the external inputs of the*

*world. Some people swing in their cycles to the point of
creating illness in themselves and in the others around
them.*

Current research indicates that as many as 50 percent of all women in
the childbearing years may suffer from PMS (pre-menstrual
syndrome). This is now treated with the male hormone progesterone,
which balances the female hormone estrogen. This balancing makes
the woman biochemically more *androgynous* and relieves the
symptoms of excessive tension and irrationality.

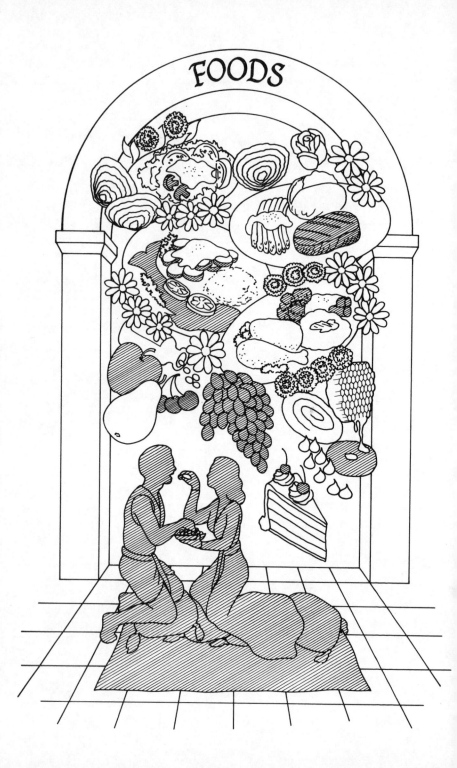

*The first and foremost erogenous zone
is in the mind.*

Foods

Emotional symptoms that affect our attitudes and energy in bed may be part of a metabolic problem and may be curable by simple dietary measures. The *anxiety reaction,* most common of the "bedroom problems," occurs when the medula part of the adrenal glands responds to emotional stress by pumping out *adrenaline,* which in turn raises blood sugar. It also increases blood pressure and heart rate. The body releases adrenaline to help you "cope." An outpouring of adrenaline is the body's corrective mechanism for falling blood sugar. Many people get panic attacks for no apparent reason, and this may simply be caused by low blood sugar. Such a reaction is *hypoglycemic.* Due to our "civilized" diet and lifelong exposure to junk food, we now have a hyper-responsive insulin mechanism.

After one has indulged in refined carbohydrates, this hyper-responsive insulin mechanism responds by dropping the blood sugar to a point below that at which it started. The body must then call upon the same adrenaline mechanism to raise the blood sugar to normal. In this case the same symptoms that come with an anxiety attack appear, without the stress of something ominous to touch things off.

Since the levels of insulin and adrenaline are major biochemical correlates with anxiety symptoms and respond to blood sugar changes, *the controlling of blood sugar is an important key to controlling anxiety.* An increase of serotonergic activity in the brain accompanies the pancreatic secretions of insulin during the assimilation of a meal, especially one rich in carbohydrates. This increase is directly related to the subjective experience of drowsiness, which commonly follows a meal.

Ingestion of dietary fats, or the metabolism of stored body fats during a fast, is known to cause an excess of brain serotonin as the result of increased availability of free tryptophan. The trophotropic function is said to be responsible for the accumulation of tension, while the ergotropic mediates the release of these energies.

All physiological systems need a rest. At the molecular level, this is evident in the dynamics of drugs and drug receptors. Too excessive a use of "europhenigenic" drugs prevents the experience of euphoria from occurring. The system begins to require more and more of the drug, until eventually no amount of the drug will produce the desired effect.

A treatment for sluggish digestive enzymes involves short fasts and daily dietary rotation of different food groups. This allows some of the enzyme systems to "rest" while others are active.

General health influences sexual health. The condition of our nerves, blood, arteries, heart, muscle tone, and digestion can greatly determine our abilities in bed. Our sexuality is not merely in our gonads. It permeates every cell in our bodies. A pronounced lack of one of the vitamin or mineral groups is often the cause of reduced sexual desire and performance. Here is a list of vitamins and minerals that appear to influence human sexuality.

Vitamin A—This vitamin has been called nature's shield against glandular stress. Ample intake is required against the possibility of sterility. Vitamin A has a protective effect on the adrenal glands. Not only does it prevent adrenal enlargement, but it also blocks the shrinkage of the thymus gland. It works hand-in-hand with Vitamin E. If you are taking large quantities of E, you should also take 25,000 units of A. Unsaturated fatty acids (sometimes called Vitamin F) are necessary for the proper assimilation of A and E. Together, they are needed for normal gland activity and have been used to treat prostate and menstrual disorders.

Vitamin B_1 (thiamine)—It has been called the morale vitamin, and its lack can result in almost any nervous manifestation you can name. Thiamine deficiencies can set moods swinging. B_1 is needed to convert body fuels into energy. Deficiency soon results in fatigue, depression, anxiety, and apathy. Like all B-complex vitamins, thiamine must be consumed daily. All excess is excreted. (R.D.A.: 1.5 milligrams.)

Vitamin B_2 (riboflavin)—Studies show that when the body is deprived of riboflavin, adrenal exhaustion develops, accompanied by hemorrhaging of the glands. It is a marked cause of depression. It is necessary for healthy skin and tissue and for the protection of the eyes from glare. The best sources are liver, dark, green vegetables, milk, eggs, and wheat germ. It is the most commonly deficient vitamin in our diets. (R.D.A.: 1.7 mgs.)

Vitamin B_3 (niacin)—One of the early signs of niacin depletion is the loss of a sense of humor. It is necessary for the metabolism of carbohydrates and promotes proper functioning of the nervous system, as well as brain and blood circulation. The body can manufacture some of its own niacin with the help of tryptophan (present in milk and protein foods). The best sources are liver, lean meats, milk, eggs, and dried yeast. Too high a dose of niacin will cause flushing, itching of the skin, and a feeling of intense heat. (R.D.A.: 19 mgs)

Vitamin B₅ (pantothenic acid) — B₅ aids in metabolizing carbohydrates, proteins, and fats. It fortifies white blood cells. When depleted, it can result in profound depression and lowered resistance to stress. It is found in whole-grain cereals, chicken, pork, liver, and kidneys. It is also associated with hair becoming grey, although that research is inconclusive.

Vitamin B₆ (pyridoxine) — B₆ promotes healthy teeth, gums, and skin. It also assists in the manufacture of hemoglobin and certain hormones. The best sources are liver, bananas, lima beans, potatoes, whole-grain cereals, and brewer's yeast. It may also prevent excessive fluid retention. (R.D.A.: 2.2 mgs)

Vitamin B₁₂ (cyanocobalamin) — It is essential for the formation of red blood cells. Its deficiency can lead to nervous system degeneration and loss of energy. Only animal products such as eggs, liver, kidneys, beef, and milk can supply B₁₂. Strict vegetarian diets may risk a deficiency resulting in anemia, loss of balance, and pain and weakness in the arms and legs. Brewer's yeast and spiralina are excellent vegetable sources of B₁₂. (R.D.A.: 0.2 mgs)

Vitamin B₁₅ (pangamic acid) — Its function is to bring oxygen to all the tissues. Because of this it helps to prevent premature impotence and most degenerative diseases. Yeast products are quite good as a source of B₁₅, although the richest source by far for this vitamin is the kernel of the apricot.

Vitamin B₁₇ (amygdalin or laetrile) — Little is known about this vitamin. Some believe that it destroys cancer cells without harming normal tissue. Chemically, laetrile is a cyanide molecule safely sandwiched between two other molecules. Our bodies, however, produce an enzyme (rhodanese) which neutralizes metabolic cyanide before it can harm the tissues. This vitamin is also derived from the kernels of apricots, where it occurs naturally and in abundance. It has also been shown to be an effective contraceptive. Papaya seeds are actually eaten by Polynesian women just for this purpose. They use twenty-five seeds per day.

Biotin—This is necessary for the metabolism of carbohydrates. It helps maintain the sweat glands, blood cells, and skin. It also helps maintain thyroid and adrenal glands. It is needed to break down foods. The best sources are eggs, green vegetables, liver, and milk. A true biotin deficiency is rare. (R.D.A.: 0.2 mgs)

Folic acid (folacin)—This helps the body produce antibodies against infection and maintains functions in the lower intestinal tract. Deficiency has been linked to some mental disorders. It is best found in leafy, green vegetables, fruits, dried peas and beans, and wheat germ. (R.D.A.: 60 mgs)

Vitamin C (ascorbic acid)—This is essential for healthy adrenal glands, the glands containing the highest concentration of Vitamin C. The pituitary gland demands daily or near daily supplies of this water-soluble substance for proper functioning. The vitamin also buffers the system against general debility, which in itself could have an effect on the sexual system. The best sources are citrus fruits, berries, cabbage, tomatoes, and potatoes. Vitamin C must be consumed daily, as it helps protect against unwanted oxidation of other vitamins. (R.D.A.: 60 mgs)

Vitamin D—This vitamin is required for the proper assimilation of calcium and phosphorus. It is produced by the body through exposure to sunlight *(calciferol)*.

Vitamin E (mixed tocopherols)—There are over 100 related compounds from the tocopherol group, with alpha-tocopherol being the most active compound in the series. It is found in greatest concentration in the anterior pituitary gland, where it positively influences the production of male sex hormones. It also protects these hormones and other vital substances in the body from oxidation. It helps to break up accumulations of arterial cholesterol and to conserve oxygen in the blood. Doses of 400 to 1,600 units daily can be taken without side effects. Oil-soluble vitamins are best taken after a large meal containing fats or oils. *Persons suffering from extreme high blood pressure or heart damage from chronic rheumatic fever should not take large amounts of Vitamin E.* Women on oral contraceptives require greater amounts of folic acid and Vitamin E.

Lecithin—There is a larger proportion of lecithin in the brain, central nervous system, and seminal fluids than in any other parts of the body. It must be replaced after orgasm. Good sources are unrefined vegetable oils, unroasted seeds or nuts, and eggs. This substance increases the quality and quantity of the spermatozoa.

Linoleic acid—This substance appears to be able to help preserve youthfulness.

Iron—This mineral helps to maintain good general health and keeps the sexual system in condition.

Magnesium—A deficiency of this mineral can adversely affect the production of semen in the male. Fruits, vegetables, whole-grain breads, wheat germ, and nuts and seeds are good sources of this mineral. It is also important in reproduction and in the proper function of the mammary glands.

Nucleic acid—Although little is still known about this compound, it seems to keep grey hair from forming. It also vitalizes the body and thus promotes keener sexual enjoyment.

Phosphorus—This mineral seems to be absolutely necessary in promoting normal sexual desire and activity. Heavy doses almost invariably lead to increased erotic interest, with total absence from the system affecting semen production. Combined with calcium the body is assured of better absorption.

Postassium—This mineral increases muscular tone and glandular strength and thus helps to ward off fatigue. A severe deficiency of this mineral can cause depression of the libido, kidney and prostate problems, and other problems related to stroke and heart conditions. It is found in figs, canteloupes, bananas, avacados, and vinegar.

Zinc—This mineral plays an important role in the growth and maturity of the male sexual organs. Deficiencies result in unhealthy changes in the structure and size of the prostate gland. More zinc is found in the male reproductive system than anywhere else in the body. The highest concentrations are found in the prostate and seminal fluids, with the most in the sperm cells. A zinc deficiency can interfere with male sexual prowess. The consumption of snails and oysters, which contain large concentrations of zinc, was recommended in previous times to improve sexual performance. Some of the best sources are nuts, seeds (especially pumpkin, sunflower, and sesame seeds), liver, and yeast.

Good nutrition is an extremely important part of optimum fitness. All too often we do not pay much attention to what goes into our bodies. The food we eat is the fuel for our system and supplies us with energy. Eating the right foods can help sexual tone and desire, as well as provide nutrients to the tissues. A well-balanced diet includes foods found in the four basic food groups.

1. *Milk Group:* These supply protein, calcium, and riboflavin. Foods in this group are cheeses, cottage cheese, and milk or ice cream. The minimum daily requirement is two or more servings of milk or its equivalent.

2. *Bread/Cereal Group:* These supply carbohydrates, iron, and the B vitamins (thiamin, niacin, and riboflavin). These are found in barley, rye, wheat, corn, oats, rice, buckwheat, and grits. The minimum daily requirement is four servings.

3. *Vegetable/Fruit Group:* These supply Vitamins A and C and some iron. These are found in green, leafy (light and dark) vegetables, citrus fruits, potatoes, squashes, cabbage, and peppers. The minimum daily requirement is citrus fruit (for Vitamin C) and dark green or deep yellow vegetables 3 to 4 times weekly (for Vitamin A).

4. *Meat Group:* These supply protein, iron, B vitamins, and other minerals (phosphorus). Foods in this group are beef, veal, pork, lamb, wild game, fish and shellfish, poultry, eggs, legumes, and nuts. The minimum daily requirement is two or more servings.

In themselves, these different food groups are not aphrodisiacs or virility enhancers. But, inasmuch as they contain the vitamins, minerals, enzymes, and amino acids necessary for good health, they can sharpen the sexual tone of the body.

Ritual Use

Good sex and good food have always gone well together. The art of kissing probably stems from mouth-to mouth feeding. Even with current studies, sexual responsiveness in women was "positively and significantly correlated wiht their general positive attitude toward food and eating." Like sex, you should take time together when you eat, relaxing and not rushing things.

To ritualize a meal is to lend grace and style to the action of eating. It is a method of organizing the experience. The manner in which the meal is "perceived" will determine the possible ways in which the specific symbolism may be incorporated into our daily lives. By creating this "sacred time" via a ritual, new meaning is given to a meal.

The best-known ritual with a food is the Japanese Tea Ceremony. Because of the intricate patterns (or forms) in the ritual, it takes time to perform. It also adds a very special type of meaning when you wish to give a formal greeting to a friend. This ritual is given as a model to use in creating your own methods of spending more "sacred time" with your lover. It is only one of many rituals that can be done with food.

Since earliest times tea has been used by Buddhist monks to keep their minds alert during the long hours of meditation. Gradually, the method of preparing and sipping it became a ritualized sequence of movements, a formal dance of significant gestures designed to purge the mind of irrelevant concerns and establish a state of tranquil, alert receptivity free from normal day-to-day occurences.

In one of the oral traditions of the Chinese Ch'an Buddhist religious rites, the monks drank tea out of a single bowl while standing in front of the image of Bodhidharma. Awestruck by the splendor of the early T'ang court, the Japanese attempted to imitate these artistic styles. What eventually emerged was the *Cha-no-yu,* or "hot-water tea" ceremony (1477).

The tea ceremony was the ritualized formula for the serving of tea by a host to five or less guests. It was considered an interval of meditation and aestheticism. The ceremony was held in a tea room, a room separated from an ordinary Japanese house. Later, the tea room became an element in a special building known as the tea house. This house consisted of a tea room (designed to hold fewer than six persons), an anteroom where tea utensils were washed and stored, a waiting room for the guests, and a garden path connecting the waiting room to the tea room.

The elements of the tea house were devised and interpreted according to Zen philosophy. For example, the garden path signified the first stage of meditation, the passage into self-illumination. Built as artistic showplaces, the tea houses were carefully constructed so as to seem natural and unselfconscious. The entire ceremony was intended as a work of art.

The famous tea master Sen-no Rikyu first created the independent tea house and formulated rules for the tea ceremony.

1. As soon as the guests were assembled in the waiting room, they announced themselves by knocking on a wooden gong.

2. It was important on beginning this ceremony to have not only a clean face and hands but also a clean heart.

3. The host must greet his guests and conduct them into the tea room. If the guests were not pleased with the service, they were to leave at once.

4. As soon as the water made boiling sounds (like the wind in the fir trees), the bell should ring. This was considered the "right moment" for the water and the fire.

5. It was forbidden to speak of anything worldly during this ritual. The only thing to be held in mind was the tea and the tea ceremony.

6. No guest or host should, in any true, pure meeting, flatter the other with either word or deed.

7. A meeting should not last longer than two hours.

The formal tea ceremony is a ritual of great exclusiveness. Each guest should carefully select dress for the occasion, avoiding ostentation., After the guests have assembled in the waiting room, the host comes to stand in the doorway and bows to greet the guests. He then returns to the tea room without saying a word. The guests follow him out of the waiting room, down a garden path to the tea room.

En route they are expected to commune with nature. They pass a stone basin full of water and wash themselves, according to the purification rites. They enter the tea room through a low door. Each guest kneels in front of a small alcove to admire a hanging scroll, which later will be replaced by a floral arrangement. They then admire the tiny incense holder on a side shelf.

Sometimes a *kaiseki* meal is served to the guests at this time. The meal is served entirely by the host, and the guests must eat everything. When the meal is over, the guests put their empty dishes and bowls on separate trays which the host removes one by one. The guests return to the waiting room, where they remain until a gong is sounded. This is the signal for them to come back to the tea room for the ceremonial tea.

When they return they notice that a flower arrangement has replaced the scroll in the tea-room alcove. The fresh-water vessel, or *mizusashi,* and the tea caddy, *cha-ire,* are already in place. When the guests are seated, the host enters with the tea bowl, tea whisk *(chasen),* tea cloth *(cha- kin),* and teaspoon *(cha-shaku).* He puts them down, leaves, then returns with the waste-water receptacle *(koboshi),* dipper *(hishaku),* and stand for the kettle cover and dipper *(fataoki).*

The guests listen to the sound of water boiling in the kettle over the charcoal hearth recessed into the floor. After they have commented on the kettle, tea is prepared. This is done by placing three spoonsful of tea into the bowl. The bowl is filled with hot water. The dipper used for this purpose is returned to the kettle into which any excess water is poured. Both are then put aside. The host stirs the tea with the whisk until it becomes frothy. He then hands the tea bowl to the principal guest, who bows to his fellow guests and sips the tea. He should then compliment the host and sip again from the bowl. It is then passed to the next guest.

The last person in the circle finishes the tea, always leaving a small amount in the bowl. Then the bowl, tea caddy, and spoon are passed around for the guests to admire. This tea ceremony set standards of refinement for the arts, literature, and everyday life. It has instilled in the Japanese a taste for simplicity, harmony, and balance. The ceremony is like an improvised drama whose plot is woven about the tea, the utensils, the flowers, and the paintings of the room.

The Japanese ritualized the subtle properties of tea drinking that the Chinese only appreciated instinctively. Tenuous connections between tea and connoisseurship were firmly realized in the Japanese Tea Ceremony.

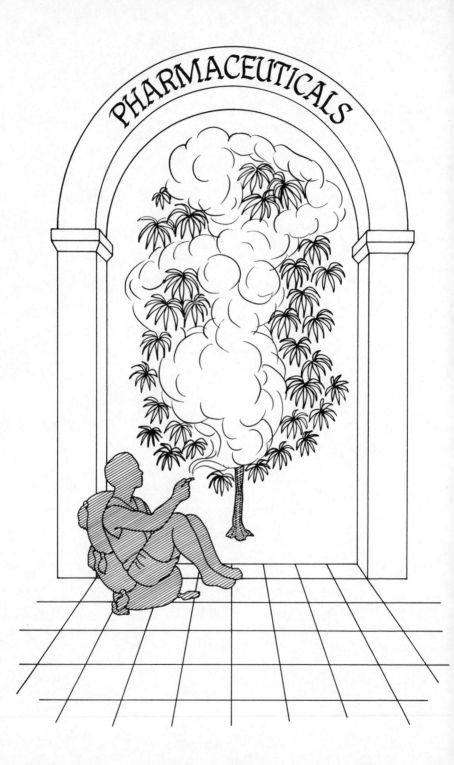

Pharmaceuticals

Most people are not aware of the fact that, to a greater or lesser extent, our love relationships are "addictive" behavior habits. They resemble amphetamine-like compounds and opiates, which lure us together, arouse sexual desire, and keep partners in pair-bonded states of attraction long after any "flames of passion" have cooled. These are the naturally occurring narcotics in our bodies known as *endorphins* and *enkephalins* (depending on their size). They act primarily as anti-anxiety agents.

The naturally occurring amphetamine-like substances are *phenylethylamine* (PEA), *norepinephrine,* and *dopamine.* They all increase with happy moods, and lower moods indicate a decrease of these chemistries in the brain. Chocolate contains PEA and several related compounds. This probably explains why the candy bar is so popular with the lovelorn.

The hypothalamus is the real chemical boss in the body. No bigger than a pea, this incredible site in the brain receives input from all parts of the body and transmits instructions to the pituitary in the form of chemicals called releasing factors. These substances stimulate the pituitary to release its various hormones. These, in turn, affect the sex glands' production of hormones—estrogen and progesterone in the female ovaries and androgens from the Leydig's cells of the male testes.

There are two vital neuropathways in this system. The first connects the hypothalamus to the pituitary and tells it when to release hormones. The second connects the hypothalamus to the higher thinking and knowing part of the brain. This area tells us when to initiate appropriate mating behavior. The most interesting hypothalamic chemical discovered to date is called LHRH (luteinizing-hormone releasing hormone).

LHRH seems to be responsible for synchronizing the behavioral and endocrinological aspects of mating. It produces sexual arousal of the brain prior to ovulation, when the female is most receptive to impregnation (in animals). It now appears that humans can produce this at will; this allows them to engage in sex all the time, irrespective of reproductive considerations or seasonal changes.

The state associated with feelings of "falling in love" is very similar to an amphetamine boost. With continued intimacy, however, the novelty of the relationship wears off, and those initial feelings of elation give way to new emotions. These are the emotions that cement the tie between partners. It is these two phases of romance—attraction and attachment—which are now believed to be determined primarily by biology.

There are two distinct neurochemical systems, the amphetamine-like compounds and the opiates. The opiates are narcotics that suppress the activity of the *locus ceruleus,* which is involved in producing such things as anxiety and panic. MAO (monoamine oxidase) enzymes are the most important of the brain enzymes, helping the body to break down by oxidation (metabolize) chemical substances called monoamines. These substances include the amphetamine-like compounds of PEA, norepinephrine, dopamine, and serotonin. These MAO enzymes help regulate the number of important transmitters available for brain activity at any given moment.

Lower MAO activity means greater amounts of brain monoamines. Thus, the first true antidepressant drug, *iproniazid,* was an *MAO inhibitor.* Lower MAO levels are thus associated with higher sensation-seeking responses. At a neurochemical level, attachment is essentially an addictive phenomenon involving opioids, the brain's version of opiates. A dependence on these opioids is what fosters the close ties between a mother and her infant. These same chemistries bond a man and a woman.

It is this method of pair-bonding that helps partners stay together, at least long enough to conceive and raise children. *While it is the amphetamine-like compounds which bring people together through attraction, it is the opioids which keep them together.* We have all known what most refer to as the "attachment junky," a person who needs to be with another person at all times. Their biochemical makeup produces too few opioids, so they have a tendency to cling to their mates. This almost instinctual behavior is an attempt to keep the level in their neural reservoirs from falling below some threshold mark. Essentially they are using their partners as mood regulators.

Autism, on the other hand, may be, in part, a result of overproduction of these opioids. A surplus of opioids would make an individual not bond to the mother or feel a need for physical affection, something commonly seen in autistic children.

With these perspectives, it is quite easy to see that when one breaks a relationship, the resulting emotional trauma seems very similar to a drug withdrawal. It may thus be postulated that a "longing of the heart" is most often a form of addiction.

The following list of pharmaceuticals may contain substances that are illegal in the United States and Europe. Others have restrictions or may soon be outlawed. They are listed because they have attracted considerable interest among the public. Although this section describes various ways to use them, this should not be construed as encouragement or endorsement by the author or publisher.

This section is written in the belief that you have a right to information and knowledge even when these

151

pharmaceuticals have the potential for abuse. It is our hope that with this information, the reader will learn how to avoid the abuse of the drugs described. Furthermore, we are not prescribing any of the substances, legal or otherwise, to the reader. Therefore, we can in no way be held responsible for any mishaps or failures that may occur through the use or misuse of any of these materials or this information.

Alcohol *(Ethanol)*—Alcohol acts as a sexual stimulant for many people when utilized in small quantities. It depresses the brain centers that govern fear, thus reducing anxiety. Small doses such as those occasioned by social drinking release inhibitions sufficiently to often cause a temporary increase in libido, especially in inhibited persons. It reverses its chemical reaction when taken in larger doses or for a long period of time. Long-term usage as a sexual stimulant turns it into a sexual depressant which will definitely diminish the libido instead of elevating it.

Amyl Nitrate—This drug is a vasodilator which is sometimes prescribed to relieve the pain of angina pectoris victims and relieve certain types of asthma attacks. It is sold in small glass ampules which must be broken open and inhaled. The usual medical dose is 0.2 ml. The effects last for a few moments. During this time it also breaks down inhibitions in much the same manner as nitrous oxide (laughing gas), as it works as a smooth muscle relaxant.

It is also used at the moment of climax to lengthen and intensify orgasm. It is used most often by the gay set, frequently to facilitate the penetration of the anus with the penis or hand. There are usually no unpleasant after effects, although the odor is somewhat reminiscent of rotting apples or pears. When the FDA banned its use, amyl was quickly replaced by *butyl nitrate,* which smells like old tennis shoes and is sold legally as a "room odorizer."

Amyl nitrate has hypotensive (blood pressure decrease) effects. Because of this it may be dangerous when used by persons suffering from low blood pressure. Side effects include headaches and, in rare cases, heart attacks.

Cannabis (Cannabis sativa and *Cannabis indica*)— Also known as marijuana, the Chinese have made use of this as a medicinal plant for at least 5,000 years. The earliest use of marijuana was by the Hindu peoples of India prior to 1,000 B.C. Sweetmeats were made from cannabis seeds and leaves and were combined with musk and honey to create an effective concoction. (Musk is the sexual attractant produced in the glandular sac beneath the abdominal skin of the male musk deer.)

Cannabis contains tetrahydrocannabinol (THC) and cannibichrome. It also contains antibiotics and sedatives such as cannabigerol and cannabidiolic acid. They mostly function as a sedative, *not* as a narcotic. It relaxes the mind and body, diminishes unnecessary inhibitions, and opens one to sensual awareness. Women are more likely to report an increase in desire, while men usually report an increase in the enjoyment of sex.

The African aphrodisiac *Khala-Khif* is made from normal marijuana that has been fortified with extracted resins. A blue mold forms and is allowed to work on the mixture for approximately one month. The resulting powerful product is then dried and smoked. This form is similar to hashish (the resinous extract gathered from the tops of the plant) or hash oil (any refinement or concentrate derived from the crude extracts).

Coca *(Erthroxylon coca)*—Cocaine is one of the several alkaloids found in this South American shrub. The leaves of the coca bush have a long history of enthusiastic usage. The Indians in Ecuador, Bolivia,

153

and Brazil chew the leaf with a little banana ash or some other mild caustic such as slaked lime. Two ounces of leaves taken in this manner release over 1/2 gram of cocaine into the body.

A snort or two through the nostrils permits arousal of the libido and a more sustained sexual act than is normally possible. A man who has taken cocaine may find himself maintaining an erection even after one or more orgasms. The drug also tends to give a man great control over orgasm. Occasionally, however, the drug will so greatly stimulate the intellectual centers that the individual can be distracted from sensual desire to the extent that all the person may want to do is think or talk out their thoughts.

People who are into kinky forms of sex (offbeat, unusual, or even bizarre sexual experimentation) find cocaine the ideal drug to put them in the mood for such pleasures. Applied topically as a surface anesthetic, a little cocaine on the clitoris will anesthetize the surface irritation and enable the woman to enjoy many more orgasms. It has also been applied to the head and shaft of the penis to decrease sensation and prevent premature ejaculation.

Cocaine is also now considered quite addictive, with numerous horror stories of its abuse. Excessive snorting of cocaine can do damage to the nasal membranes and olfactory nerves. Its possession and use is also a Class A felony.

DMSO *(Dimethyl sulfoxide)*—DMSO is a solvent substance derived from wood pulp as a byproduct of the paper industry. It has the unusual property of being swiftly absorbed through the skin into the blood stream. It may also, in some cases, carry other substances with it into the blood. A dab of DMSO on the penis can often produce a quick erection in cases of impotence. It should not be taken internally and even when used topically can have damaging effects upon the kidneys if used in large quantities. It seems to be

154

non-toxic when used externally in small doses.

L-Dopa *(levo-rotary isomer of dihydroxyphenyl-alanine)*—Also known as levodopa or Larodopa (trade mark of Roche Laboratories), it is primarily used in the treatment of Parkinson's disease. It also causes increased sexual desire in most individuals. In some cases it may have some very undesirable side effects, including nausea, anxiety, depression, confusion, lethargy, blurred vision, hot flashes, and hair loss.

It should not be taken by persons who are currently taking MAO inhibitors or by pregnant or lactating mothers. Others who should avoid L-dopa include persons with an active peptic ulcer or those who are taking antihypertensive drugs. It is only available by a prescription. It is a serotonin inhibitor and like most other psychedelics (including LSD, psilocybin, mescaline, DMT, yage', and yohimbe) is a mild hallucinogen.

MDA *(Methylenedioxyamphetamine)*— Known as the "love drug," this is probably the only psychedelic drug with a clear reputation for increasing libido. MDA is an amphetamine-related hallucinogen with effects that are truly sexually stimulating. If the MDA you find is real, you probably want to do nothing but make love for the following four or five hours. Most people use doses of 120 to 150 mg to obtain the full range of effects.

About thirty to sixty minutes after ingestion, depending on the thickness of the capsule, some nausea usually occurs. There are none of the perceptual distortions or closed-eye imagery triggered by such drugs as LSD, but there is a heightening of visual acuity. Objects appear brighter and sharper than normal. Most striking are the intensified feelings and empathy with others. These effects can persist for up to eight hours, but the peak of the experience comes about two hours after ingestion.

The most common adverse effect is a periodic tensing of neck and jaw muscles. The main problem with the use of MDA is that the substance usually purchased on "the streets" is not MDA but something much more toxic (like PCP, also known as "angel dust").

Methaqualone *(2-methyl-3-o-tolyl-4(3H)-quinazolinone)*—Sold under the name Quaalude, Sopor, Parrest, and Mandrax, this drug is a sedative and hypnotic agent. The drug works as do alcohol and cocaine, releasing normal inhibitions. It appears to act upon a different central nervous system site than the barbiturates and other hypnotic drugs. Tolerance to quaaludes develops quite rapidly and can lead to addiction.

Many women who ordinarily lack interest and energy for sex become much more interested in erotic pleasure after taking this drug. Usual dosage ranges from 150 to 300 mg for sleep, with 75 to 150 mg prescribed to combat nervousness for daytime sedation. Driving while under the influence is quite dangerous, and some experience hangovers accompanied by blurred thinking and vision. It must not be taken in combination with alcohol as it can be fatal.

Opium Poppy *(Papaver somniferum)*—Although opium, the dried latex-like exudate of the poppy, is a narcotic, it can be an erotic aphrodisiac when taken moderately. It has a stimulating effect upon the spinal ganglia, producing an erection similar to that of strychnine, yohimbe, and burra gokeroo *(Pedalium murex)*. It has a relaxing and sedating effect upon the body and mind in general but it stimulates erotic feelings on both the mental and physical levels.

These sensations can be increased by using it as a mild anesthetic for the surface nerves of the sex glands in both males and females. This delays ejaculation and allows the development, during sex, of the deeper stimulation of underlying nerves. This tends to prolong the sexual act, and a sexual climax may become a more intense and more psychic experience. Like most other narcotics, however, excessive use can weaken one's sexual powers.

Various narcotic drugs have been used as sexual aids for centuries. These include the natural drugs such as morphine, alcohol, and nicotine. Synthetic and semi-synthetics such as meperidine (Demerol), dihydromorphine (Dilaudid), and methadone (Dolaphine) are also part of this list. They are all also very addictive. Many people become nauseous shortly after the ingestion of opium.

Pemoline   *(2-imino-5-phenyl-4-oxazolidinone)* — Pemoline was used by American and British flyers during World War II to maintain alertness during long bombing runs. While the Nazis used amphetamines, pemoline was considered far safer and did not have the dangerous and unpleasant side effects of the latter, namely cardiac stress, drying of mucous membranes, tension in neck and facial muscles, and an addictive potential. It is a synthetically prepared hydantoin group chemical. The usual dose (20 to 50 mg orally) gives mental stimulation lasting for six to twelve hours.

It is combined with yohimbine hydrochloride, methyltestosterone, and strychnine sulfate in a prescriptive medicine for the temporary treatment of impotence. The mixture is marketed in England as Potensan Forte by Medo Chemicals (Archway, North London). Another form of pemoline, called pemoline magnesium, is produced in the United States (Abbott Laboratories) and has been used to improve memory and to treat senility.

Pemoline magnesium's effects are similar to the amphetamines, with smaller doses acting as a mild CNS and psychic stimulant. In this form, it causes the accumulation of magnesium in the cerebral synapses. Magnesium acts as a catalyst conductor in the synapses of the brain's memory centers. It is an excellent aphrodisiac in this form.

157

Strychnine *(Strychnos nux vomica)*—The active alkaloid strychnine is obtained from the seed of a tree from China, Burma, India, and Australia. It is effective as a stimulant and general tonic especially when combined with other substances. It has also been used as a remedy for neuralgia, dyspepsia, debility, chronic constipation, and impotence. Its action in the latter case is effected by stimulation of the circulation, the muscular system, and the spinal nerves.

Strychnine can have such a profound influence on the spinal ganglia (which controls the erectile tissue) that a man may suffer from a powerful and painful erection. It also develops strong body heat and perspiration. There is a narrow margin between an effective and a dangerous dose. Two mg can serve as a sexual stimulant, but larger amounts can cause rapid heart and pulse rates, convulsions, and even death. Individual tolerances vary. Medical supervision is absolutely recommended when using this drug. There are other substances, like yohimbe, which have a similar action but are infinitely safer to use. Essentially, strychnine lowers the synaptic jump potential between neurons in the brain. A slight lowering increases intelligence, but larger degrees of lowering these potentials produce seizures and even death. Crude extracts of *Strychnos* seeds are used in a number of preparations, including *Aphrodex* (see Yohimbe).

This list of drugs and their effects is by no means comprehensive. A book-length treatment would be needed to fully explore this topic. If you suffer from impaired self-confidence, however, a drug such as cocaine, which increases self-confidence and improves the user's self-image, might materially improve your sexual performance.

If, however, you are nervous, apprehensive, or quite inhibited when it comes to sex, small amounts of a depressant such as alcohol can loosen your inhibitions and help you relax enough to enjoy sex. Whatever contributes to healthy human functioning generally contributes specifically to enhancing libido and sexual response. And, whatever impairs healthy human functioning impairs libido and sexual response.

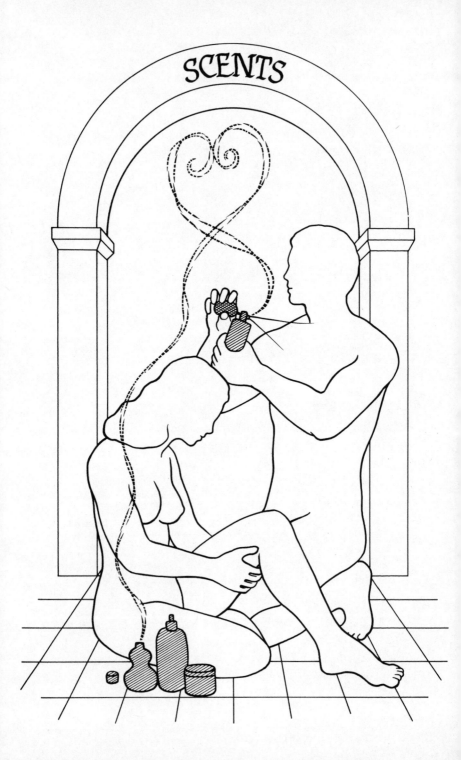

Scents

No matter how we scrub and clean ourselves, we all still emit a unique and individual odor. Furthermore, we are all profoundly affected by other people's odors and by those from our environment. No aspect of our behavior is immune from this. We communicate with a silent, invisible, often subliminal smell language whether at work, in the dining room, or at home in our bedroom.

Odors and the Brain

Smell is mediated by *olfactory receptors* in the *olfactory organ*. Axons of the olfactory receptors enter the skull and go directly to a portion of the brain known as the *olfactory bulb*. Fibers from the bulb are part of a widespread and diffuse system in the brain known as the *rhinencephalon* (from the Greek for "nose brain"). The sense of smell is actually an *exposed* portion of the brain that samples the external world as brain cells outside the skull.

Neuroanatomists have found the olfactory system to be unique because instead of going through the dorsal thalamus where the other senses establish relay stations to the neocortex (That "new" part of the

161

brain that gives us our intellect), the olfactory cells send their fibers directly to the brain area formerly called the rhinencephalon. This part of the brain is now known as the "limbic system," a term derived from the limbus, or border, rimming the cortex of the brain. This so-called "nose brain" also deals with the regulation of motor activities and the primary drives of sex, hunger, and thirst. Evolutionists now maintain that the two cerebral hemispheres of the brain actually developed from these olfactory lobes and that as the brain became more complex, the primitive limbic system remained at the forefront, exposed to the external world.

It has a primary position, they postulate, because olfaction was the first distant receptor that could operate efficiently in a water medium like the ocean. Since life evolved from the sea, the first part of the brain to develop was that area concerned with smell. Stimulation of the olfactory bulb shoots electrical signals to an almond-shaped nugget known as the *amygdala,* an area of the limbic system concerned with visceral and behavioral mechanisms, particularly those associated with sensory and sexual functions.

These signals are then relayed from the amygdala to the brain stem, the "turnpike" that contains the interconnections between brain and body. Therefore, the electrical stimulation involved in smelling directly affects the digestive and sexual systems as well as emotional behavior. Odors produce strong emotional reactions and may be remembered many years after a single exposure. The sense of smell deteriorates with age and can be adversely affected by pollutants.

Healthy young persons can distinguish among thousands of different odors. Odor memory is less influenced by the passage of time than are auditory and visual memories. Once remembered, smells are rarely, if ever, forgotten. This is because they stir basic emotions and become associated with "feelings." Memories can be instantly recalled if you catch a whiff of an odor from your childhood: the scent your mother used; your father's after- shave lotion; your home; your classroom. We are able to take one sniff and identify a single aroma from among thousands we have experienced in our past.

In a liter of air, a person can smell as little as one four-hundred-billionth of a gram of ethyl mercaptan (essence of rotten meat). That person would have to taste considerably more before noticing it. Smell is more than ten thousand times more sensitive than taste.

The nose can also smell directionally. The small difference in odor stimuli between the two nostrils is enough to reveal the direction of an odor source. The human nose is five times more sensitive than the rat's when it comes to detecting changes in odor intensity.

Classification of Odors

There have been many attempts, dating back to the eighteenth century, to classify odors. Most scientists accepted the notion that there were six or seven basic odors: *ethereal, camphoraceous, musky, floral, minty, pungent,* and *putrid.* These odors can be organized in a space known as the *smell prism.*

This structure suggests the existence of primary odors. However, mixtures of odorous substances fail to give clear support to the idea that all odors can be mimicked by some mixture of a fundamental set of odors. Sometimes mixtures produce unitary experiences, but most often a person can distinguish the components of a compound odor.

According to the *stereochemical theory of odor,* the odor of a substance is related to the shape of its molecules. However, the odors of substances composed of small molecules are related to their chemical properties rather than their shapes. There have been numerous theories on how the brain receives and interprets information from the nose. Most can categorize these as chemical theories. These hold that molecules or particles of odorants touching the olfactory cilia are absorbed, thus creating an electrochemical change in the nose's sensory cells, which then sends electrical signals to the brain.

Some believe that enzymes, the body's catalysts, are somehow involved in the recognition and relay of odor information. Others theorize that specific odor molecules fit into specific receptors in the nose just as a round peg fits into a round hole. Dr. John Amoore (U.S.D.A. Western Regional Research Laboratory) believes that there are at least thirty primary odors. Just as we combine primary colors such as blue and yellow to make green, we combine these different odors to create the myriad of smells in our environment.

Dr. Amoore claims to have isolated four of these primary odors, three of which (isovaleric acid, 1-pyrroline, and trimethylamine) are suspected of being primate, and even human, *pheromones*. The fourth (isobutyraldehyde) occurs in a wide variety of foods. Its malty odor may signal the presence of three indispensable amino acids needed in our daily diet. The primary odors yet to be identified may provide sensory input about foods, localities, and predators. The most intriguing are problably the pheromones, the sexual scents found in living creatures.

Pheromones

The term "pheromone" is a composite from the Greek, which means literally "to transfer excitement." It was coined in 1959 by German scientists to describe the sex attractants of insects. Although pheromones were once thought to be a sex bait for insects, new evidence indicates that smell is also part of the courtship language of reptiles, birds, fish, and mammals, including primates. There are exchanges going on between a man and woman which are barely perceptible olfactory cues, even across a crowded room. The existence of human pheromones, while still in debate, has gained support with the discovery of *apocrine glands*.

Apocrine glands are narrow pits at the base of the hair follicles that produce an as yet unidentified scent chemical. Our underarm and genital hair is designed to collect this odor. As with all other mammals, human apocrines are small until puberty. The actual odors we release seem to be unique to each individual. Although quite subtle, this uniqueness in odor may account for individual preferences and pair-bonding.

The odor of trimethylamine is well known to organic chemists, who describe it as "fishy." It is formed by bacterial action on betaine, which sometimes taints the milk of cows and is most pronounced in dead fish that have not been refrigerated. There is a good deal of evidence that trimethylamine may be an important mammalian sex attractant, as well as a human pheromone.

The Swedish botanist Carolus Linnaeus noted in 1756 that the domestic dog was extremely fond of the odor of the plant *Chenopodium vulvaria*. It was given this Latin name for good reason—it smells like human menstrual blood. Its tissue contains a large amount of trimethylamine. Trimethylamine is prominent in human menstrual blood, and it is quite well-known phenomenon that the odor of mentruating women brings many male animals into a state of sexual excitation.

This suggests that trimethylamine might be a common estrus-signaling pheromone for several mammalian species. Sex pheromones are produced by both sexes. Among the pheromones identified so far among mammals, the male sex pheromones seem mainly to function as aphrodisiacs for the female, while the female sex pheromones apparently announce her sexual readiness.

There may be debate about human susceptibility to pheromones, but external chemical messengers—odors —have been shown to penetrate the human subconscious. Within seconds after exposure to an unnoticed olfactory stimulus, the electrical resistance of the person's skin decreases, and changes occur in blood pressure, respiration, and pulse rate. It is assumed that a volatile chemical, not necessarily detected as an odor, causes changes in the brain.

History

More than 5,000 years ago, Egyptians burned a a number of sweet-smelling fragrances to the sun god, Ra, as he made his daily journey across the sky. The Egyptians also used perfumes for anointing their favored and embalming their dead. They taught their art of perfumery to the slaves, the Hebrews, who then recorded the use of many aromatic materials in their sacred books. When the Hebrews left Egypt, they took with them the knowledge of the power of perfumes and the formulas for making certain mixtures.

In 1700 B.C., the Ishmaelites came from Gilead with their camels bearing a number of the spices and gums used in these formulas. Many are still used today in major perfume industries. The Queen of Sheba also used perfumes to conquer. When she visited Solomon, around 800 B.C., she brought him fragrances and successfully seduced him, putting yet another set of legends under the power of aromatics.

Babylon, Nineveh, and Carthage became great centers of perfumery in the seventh century B.C. The inhabitants collected aromatics from Arabia (gums), camphor from China, and cinnamon from India. These were exported by the Phoenicians to the entire world. The use of perfumes reached its zenith in 650 B.C. when the ruler Ashurbanipal dressed himself up like a woman, using cosmetics and perfumes.

The ancient Greeks learned the art of perfumery from the Asian countries. Hippocrates, the most famous of their physicians, outlined a study of the skin and advocated not only healthful living habits but also specially scented baths and massages. He also recommended perfumes as medication for certain diseases.

166

Ritual Use

Since time immemorial perfumes and sweet-smelling herbs have played an important part in both religion and sex magic. Exotic scents have charmed and lured both men and women and are part of the broader aspect known as the *alchemy of scent.*

The lore of perfume is only the outer veil, the inner mysteries having been carefully kept secret. This sacred science, known as the arcane science of perfume, is based on laws of "vibration" and "psycho-sensory" responses observed over long periods of history. A truly "magical" formula works on the subconscious mind, as well as the conscious, in order to illicit a specific predetermined response.

Specific formulas not only call forth a given response but can also condition the consciousness. It is a scientific fact that we all respond consciously and unconsciously to the "vibrations" of sound, color, and scent. Certain scents can cause us to feel or react in either an emotional or physical manner. Some scents stimulate the sexual centers in particular.

It is this science of psycho-sensory response that is behind all true magical formulas. In her book *The Arts Magian* (privately printed), Lady Sara Cunningham-Carter classifies all the various scents related to sexual response by their general planetary rulership, as well as by their individual "vibration." Research and experimentation should lead you to some exciting and rewarding discoveries.

The oils for just the planet Venus (goddess of love) are only some of the oils covered in this text and are given as:

Almond Oil, bitter *(Amygdalus amara).* Used in matters of love and friendship for its harmonious and magnetic vibrations.

Aloe-Wood Oil *(Aquilaria agallocha).* Generally mixed with musk and worn to attract love.

167

Alpine Rose Oil *(Rhododendron ferruginenum).* Worn for its magnetic properties as an aid in matters of romance and matrimony.

Ambrosia Oil *(Chenopodium ambrosioides).* A very sensual vibration, it is worn to attract a lover.

Amyris Oil *(Amyris balsamifera).* Used as a sacred anointing oil in Venusian rites. It is also used as an aid in past life recall.

Artemisia Oil *(Artemisia vulgaris).* Used in perfume blends and designed to arouse one's sexual desires. It is also said to restore lost sexual virility.

Bigonia Oil *(Bignolia suaveolens).* A fragrance of sexual enchantment, it is highly sensual and exotic.

Birch Oil, sweet *(Betula lenta).* Generally used in conjunction with other oils to formulate essences relating to love and sexual attraction.

Camellia Oil *(Camallia sasanqua).* A subtle yet haunting fragrance that will make its wearer unforgettable.

Cardamom Oil *(Elettoria cardamomum).* A very magnetic essence used for sexual attraction.

Coriander Oil *(Coriandrum sativum).* Worn as an oil of attraction, it is also said to keep a love relationship harmonious.

Cyclamen Oil *(N.O. Primulaceae).* A delicate fragrance that is said to keep love true and harmonious.

Hawthorn Oil *(Crataegus Oxycatha).* Very soothing and tranquil, it is said to heal misunderstandings and is excellent for high-strung individuals.

Laudanum Oil *(Cistus creticus L.).* A slightly narcotic-like fragrance that is very magnetic.

Lovage Oil *(Livisticum officinale).* Said to increase one's personal magnetism, it is worn as an oil of attraction.

Orris Oil *(Iris florentina).* Worn on the person to attract the opposite sex.

Rose Oil *(Rosa centifolia/Rosa damascena).* Promotes thoughts of love and affection. It has peaceful and harmonious vibrations. It may also be used as an anointing oil for devotional objects.

Vanilla Oil *(Vanilla planifolia).* Very soothing, it is used in healing and in certain "love" perfumes.

Today the nose is used to symbolize a whole range of attitudes. When we stick our nose into other people's business we are interfering. When we stick our noses up in the air we are snooty. If we thumb our noses at someone we signify rejection. And, of course, if we rub noses with someone we demonstrate affection.

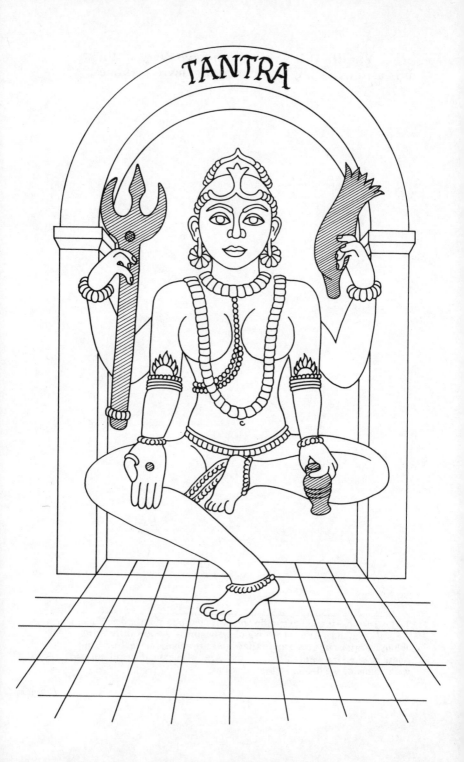

"The thought that occurs at the moment of climax happens!"

Tantra

YOGA FORMS

The word *yoga* is derived form the Sanscrit root *yog*, which means union or contact. It is, in fact, the science of the union of the human being with the divine dwelling within him. The various great mystical texts of India, such as the Bhagavad Gita, mention the following great divisions of Yoga.

Hatha Yoga — *Ha* means the moon and *tha* the sun. This is the regularization of the breath in order to modify the circulation of the prana or vital fluid in the physical body. By modifying his prana the yogi acts upon his psychic being, then on his mind, which is then modified. Thus, this is a yoga of *physical exercises,* or postures (asanas). This is essentially a Shivaist yoga.

Raja Yoga — Also known as the Royal Yoga, it begins where Hatha yoga ends. It works upon the mind with a view to directing the current of the prana. Mental concentration plays an essential part, and it is essentially a Vishnuist yoga.

171

Bhakti Yoga — This is the yoga of devotion, of love for the divine and for the guru who is its human form. This yoga is one of the most accessible to the Western mind, which is accustomed to the actions of the Christian mystic.

Karma Yoga—This is also known as the yoga of action and is subdivided into a number of other yogas. This is the yoga of duty accomplished without affection and without selfishness or self-interest. It is the great instruction of Arjuna by Krishna in the Gita, when the young prince, on the battlefield of Kurukshitra, hesitates before fighting.

Jnana Yoga — Also known as the yoga of knowledge, it is the intellectual realization of the divine that leads to an intuitive realization.

These are arbitrary classifications. Many of the various yogas are superimposed one upon another. It is important that the student have a teacher (or guru), for in using these without direction the student is liable to fall into a kind of psychic passivity, absolutely the opposite of the mystic experiences of yoga. The purpose of the teacher is to regulate the exercises and assign the method suitable to the individual disciple. In this the personal factor plays a very great part.

TANTRIC YOGA

Tantra is a spiritual method or yoga that takes into account both "inner" and "outer" realities. Derived from the root words "to expand," "weave," or "extend consciousness," tantra implies a continuity beyond the physical plane. Tantric teachings evolved in India and eventually spread to Nepal, Tibet, China, Japan, Thailand, and Indonesia.

These teachings are said to be particularly relevant in this time of materialism and narcissism since all human activities can be used as tools in the tantric path toward liberation. Tantras are texts that outline specific practices. These practices are a meditational system that aims at the experience of the highest bliss in physical and spiritual relations by cultivating the totality of one's erotic potential.

Ancient scriptures containing the mystical teachings and ritual instructions of Tantraism are called *tantras.* Briefly, they teach that earthly delights stem from the union of opposites and are achieved with an ideal partner. Such a union is said to exemplify the harmony of creation and be a step toward perfection (i.e., union with God). The power of love thus becomes central to the whole of existence.

Kama, or desire, is a creative principle that aims at the perfection of life on earth, just as the divine love that Krishna bore the shepherd girl Radha represented the cosmic energies of creation in action on earth. Among the tantric aids to meditation are mantras, sacred sounds that may be visualized as yantras, and mandalas, symbols of psychic wholeness. Various meditations for the awakening of kundalini have been given under *Ritual Use* with each herb (i.e., fo-ti-tieng, iboga, kava kava, sweet flag, and others).

The first action required by the tantric yoga is the "cleansing" of the nadis, the more highly developed nerve ganglia points in the body. These points have also been associated with chakras but are really considered "tubes" connecting the various chakra points. This purification is carried out by means of special postures of the body (asanas) and by breathing exercises (pranayama).

The mind is habituated to concentrate itself upon a point or an object, real or imaginary, so as to accustom itself to remain calm and to take absolutely "the form" which the will of the yogi wishes to impose upon it. This mental process is concentration *(dharana).* When the mind can identify itself with the divine presence in every human being, a state called *samadhi* has been reached.

Kundalini is a Sanscrit word for the normally

latent psycho-sexual power that, when awakened, ascends through the central channel of the *subtle body*. The root word "kunda" means a pool or reservoir of energy. Kundalini is likened to a coiled snake, ready to strike at any moment. When this energy is correctly directed, it can bring about cosmic consciousness and liberation.

SEX MAGIC

The alchemy described in the tantric texts is often obscure and little can be made from the jargon. The secret "door" will not open to the uninitiated without a key. Rather than the transmutation of baser metals into gold, this alchemy actually takes place within the body itself. It is a hermetic distillation from actual bodily fluids, where all the instruments and utensils used by the alchemist are provided by the body itself.

By appropriate ritual movements, the gross substance within oneself can be transformed into the subtle quintessence that can reinvigorate the physical frame. Through a series of rituals, one makes the body "glow"; this activates one's supernatural faculties and puts one in communication with any entity in the universe. This naturally presupposes a complex system of a complex system of subtle anatomy and physiology based on the chakra or plexuses of the etheric body.

All power is promised to him who can siphon the lower energy toward the upper, but this is almost impossible for the ordinary man. A tremendous need for discipline is required, discipline that is usually beyond the capacity of an average individual. A sympathetic resonance does exist between the chakras, however. By tantric methods, the kundalini can be made to blaze up through each chakra, igniting each until this stream of flame reaches the crown, or sahasrara.

A complete sex magic ritual is given under the herb Iboga'. One rite commonly celebrated in many tantric sects is known as the *chakra-puja,* or circle worship. The participants sit in a circle, implying complete mutual equality among those present. They sit in alternate sexes, male to female, with another couple in the center of the circle. A ceremonial meal consisting of wine, meat, fish, and bread is followed by a rite of sexual intercourse. These five items represent certain fundamental categories that are equated with the elements and the interior faculties of the body.

The wine symbolizes fire and the subtle draught of immortality that the tantric must learn to distill and drink. The meat symbolizes air and the bodily functions that must be brought under control. Fish represents water and the techniques of sexual occultism. The bread is the earth, or the natural environment, which must be understood and controlled. Sexual intercourse *(maithuna)* symbolizes ether, the quintessence of all the elements, and is a means to the final goal of all tantric endeavors. Through it one apprehends the ultimate reality. The sex act in its normal, gross form may occasionally bring a fleeting revelation of eternal truth, but that would be rare, as the smoke of passion usually clouds the mind. Sex as a sacred ritual unclouded by passion can, however, help you to apprehend the ultimate unity. The genuine rite can reveal being, expand consciousness, and confer true bliss. The way through pleasure *(bhukti)* can lead one to redemption *(mukti).* Sex, from this perspective, can be a way of salvation. This is the basis of the secret of tantra.

ON THE PRACTICE OF RITUAL
AND CEREMONY

There are three phases of every ritual process:

1. Separation from profane or daily life,
2. The transition stage, or twilight zone, which lies between,
3. The new order or perception of reality which occurs in the sacred time of the soul.

The in between, or twilight zone, enables a state of receptivity to be established. Ritual acts reawaken deep layers of the psyche and bring the mythological or archetypal ideas back to memory. Magic (by definition) is the transition from passivity to activity in which the will is essential. Realistic action does not follow schizophrenic magic; the fantasy is a substitute for action where the ego should be weak or even absent.

Ritual is often considered as the celebration of a myth. Myth functions as a paradigm, or model. In this school of thought, the construct of a ritual can be seen as the enactment of this myth, as the myth would be represented as the source of all action. Myth is actually a dynamic expression of the motivational power of the archetype at its core.

The main value of ritual is for the soul. Ritual can be defined as an imitation of a numinous element (or godform) in the life of the aspirant. Ritual can be seen as the outward or visible form of contact or as an epiphany with an inward or spiritual grace. It is essentially a metaphorical expression of creative imagination. The symbol always starts on the inside as a form of consciousness and is projected outward. Magical rituals contain basic elements that must appear in approximately the following sequence:

1. Setting up the circle to define a working area.

2. A form of "banishing" to clear the working area and help concentration and focusing.

3. Middle pillar exercise to bring in light and build up libido or magical potency. This helps one visualize his or her subtle body or body of light.

4. Invocation, or the "calling in", of the desired godform or attribute in an attempt at self-transformation.

5. Charging of a eucharist with the energy of the godform, and its consumption as an epiphany with the god.

6. Meditative period.

7. Banishing to return the aspirant to "normal" consciousness.

8. Closing the Temple.

These steps may be expanded to include divination, dance, dramatic scenarios, or sex magic acts. Any appropriate gestures may be added (like massage or mudras), but none of these basics can be omitted without incurring the peril of exposing the soul to random forces.

The purpose of ritual lies in its expression as an art form. Partaking in its performance is an end in itself. The spiritual import lies in the quality with which the ritual is conducted. Ritual, as symbolic action, is the enactment of mythic patterns for the sheer joy of the relationship with the archetypal dimension. Remember, *the purpose of ritual is an end in itself.* This can leave no rationale behind lusting for results.

For further information on tantric yoga, please refer to *Sexual Secrets: The Alchemy of Ecstacy,* Douglas and Slinger (Destiny Books © 1979 and *The Metaphysics of Sex,* Evola (Destiny Books) © 1983.

Biography

The Author

Richard Alan Miller is a scientist of extensive and multidimensional expertise. He did his undergraduate work in Theoretical Physics at Washington State University. His graduate work included training at M.I.T. and the University of Delaware in Solid State Physics.

He then spent over a decade working in biomedical research and development for some of the most prestigious and technologically sophisticated corporations in the United States. These included the Boeing Company, E. I. duPont de Nemours and Co., and the Department of Anesthesiology of the University of Washington.

Mr. Miller's work in Physics and Parapsychology has been published in several international journals. He also has several books in print on these subjects. He has taught Parapsychology in the Natural Sciences divisions at several universities and colleges for more than ten years. He has also taught courses in Small Farm Agriculture, with two recent books on this subject, *The Potential of Herbs as a Cash Crop* and *The Nomadic Life of the Professional Forager.*

He is one of the "new" scientists, recognizing that science should not and cannot be separated from the welfare of the human being. In 1973 he formed The

178

Beltane Corporation, a company that serves as a regional wholesaler of herbs, spices, and teas to the six western states.

The company was expanded into three further companies in 1980 to grow herbs and spices as domestic sources of supply. As a physicist he invented several critical pieces of farm machinery to assist the small farmer in harvesting and processing herbs. As an agricultural scientist he has developed specific farm plans and crop sources to compete with currently imported herbs and spices.

He is married and currently lives in Grants Pass, Oregon. He and his wife Iona, who is a Jungian psychologist, have written a series of important books in philosophy, alternative health, and self-development. His current research is on the relationship between physics and psychology. This is a continuation of his work in parapsychology on the relationship between mind and matter.

The Illustrator

Connie Nygard studied art at the Corcoran School of Art and several other schools in the Los Angeles and San Francisco Bay areas. She is currently a graphic artist and illustrator who lives in the piney woods of southern Oregon. She is working on remodeling her home in the country and teaches calligraphy and fine arts to the community.

Sources of Supply

The first question most asked when one completes reading this book is "Where can I buy these diverse *aphrodisiacs?*" Because of the international content regarding the different products, a complete list is given for sources of supply. The list includes the United States, Canada, continental Europe, Asia, Africa, and the East. For herbs of the Orient, a list of Chinese companies is also given. Several firms listed are major wholesalers for those interested in cottage industries.

UNITED STATES

Aphrodesia Products, Inc.
45 Washington St.
Brooklyn, NY 11201

Green Mountain Herbs, Inc.
4890 Pearl St.
Boulder, CO 80301

Sweethardt Herbs
Box 12602
Austin, TX 78711

Hurov's Tropical Tree Nursery
Box 10387
Oahu, HI 96813

Wilcox Drug Co.
P.O. Box 391
Boone, NC 28607

S.B. Penick and Co.
100 Church St.
New York, NY 10007

Meer Corp.
9500 Railroad Ave.
North Bergen, NJ 07047

Nature's Way Products
P.O. Box 2233
Provo, UT 84601

Star and Crescent Herbs
8551 Thys Ct.,Suite C
Sacramento, CA 95828

The Whole Herb Co.
250 E. Blithedale
Mill Valley, CA 99494

San Francisco Herb, Tea & Spice
4543 Horton St.
Emeryville, CA 94608

China Herb Co.
1053 Tenth St.
San Diego, CA 92101

Magee Fur Co.
Eolia, MO 63344

Herbarium, Inc.
11016 152nd Ave.
Kenosha, WI 53140

Botanicals International, Inc.
2550 El Presidio St.
Long Beach, CA 90810

E.L. Scott & Co.
One World Trade Center, Suite 2347
New York, NY 10048

Schonfield & Sons, Inc.
12 White St.
New York, NY 10048

CANADA

Lifestream
12411 Vulcan Way
Richmond, B.C.
CANADA V6V 1J7

Botanical Health Products
P.O. Box 88, Station N
Montreal, Quebec, CANADA

Wide World of Herbs
11 St. Catherine St. E.
Montreal 129, CANADA

Golden Bough Herb Co.
212 MacKay Ave.
North Vancouver, B.C. CANADA

EUROPE

Louis-Henry Dossi
94 Avenue de Domont
95180 Montmorency
Paris, FRANCE

Wilhelm Kramer GmbH + Co.
8721 Schwebheim Ufr.
WEST GERMANY

Verenigde Nederlandse Kruidencooperative
V.N.K. Postbus 1
Elburg, HOLLAND

Heinrich Ambrosius
2000 Hamburg 13
Mittelwag 118
P.O. Box 2563 GERMANY

E.H. Worlee & Co.
Drogen Handelgesellschaft
200 Hamburg
39 Bellevue 7-8 GERMANY

Paul Muggenburg Drogen Huas
Wandaleneg 24
D-2000 Hamburg 1, WEST GERMANY

Donck
B-2620
Hemiksem (Antwerp), BELGIUM

Laboratories Galeniques Belges
7860 Lessines
BELGIUM

Occultique
73 Kettering Road
Northampton NN1 4AW

The Sorcerer's Apprentice
4/8 Burley Lodge Road
Leeds LS6 1QP

ASIA

Medimpex
P.O. Box 126
Budapest, 5 HUNGARY

AFRICA

Ahmed Kamel
11, Talaat Harb Str
Cairo, EGYPT

Adel H. Azerfanous
5,/ ACT OR BASSILI STR
MAXAD ITA ALEX - EGYPT

EL-ADB
17 Kasr El-Nil St.
P.O. Box 2217
Cairo, EGYPT

CENTRAL & SOUTH AMERICA

Central de Drogas, S.A.
Dr. Liceaga No. 113
MEXICO 7, D.F.

Jose Asa
Morelos 110-90 Piso
MEXICO 6 D.F.

THE EAST

China National Native
82 Tung An Men St.
Peking, CHINA

Dr. Majithia
174 Samuel St.
Bombay, INDIA 9

Tsewi Corp.
2nd Fl. 67 Sung Chiang Road
P. O. Box #68-75
Taipei, Taiwan 104
REPUBLIC OF CHINA

Yoo Lee Imports & Export Co., Ltd.
P.O. Box Central 402
Seoul, KOREA

Bibliography

Anderson, M. and Savary, L., *Passages: A Guide for Pilgrims of the Mind,* Harper and Row, New York, © 1973

Boer, C., *The Homeric Hymns,* Spring Publications, Inc., Irving, TX, © 1979.

Burton, Sir Richard, *The Hindu Art of Love,* Castle Books, New York, © 1967.

Burton, Sir Richard, *The Perfumed Garden,* Castle Books, New York, © 1965.

Caldwell, W., *Organic Chemistry,* Houghton Mifflin Co., Cambridge, MA, © 1943.

Conway, D., *Magic, An Occult Primer,* Bantam Books, New York, © 1973.

Crow, W., *The Occult Properties of Herbs,* Samuel Weiser, Inc., New York, © 1969.

Crowley, A., *Magick in Theory and Practice,* Lecram Press, Paris, © 1929.

Crowley, A., *Liber Aleph,* Level Press, San Francisco, © 1974.

Crowley, A., *On Magick,* Level Press, San Francisco, © 1974.

Culling, L., *The Complete Magick Curriculum of the Secret Order G:.B:.G:.,* Llewellyn Publications, St. Paul, MN, © 1971.

Culling L., *A Manual of Sex Magick,* Llewellyn Publications, St. Paul, MN, © 1971.

Cunningham-Carter, Lady Sara, *The Arts Magian,* Privately Printed (Oregon), © 1974.

Cutting, W., *Handbook of Pharmacology,* Meredith Corp., New York, © 1972.

Douglas N. and Slinger, P., *Sexual Secrets,* Destiny Books, New York, © 1979.

Emboden, W., *Narcotic Plants,* The Macmillan Co., New York, © 1972.

Evola, J., *The Metaphysics of Sex,* Inner Traditions, New York, © 1983.

Farrar, S., *What Witches Do,* Coward, McCann & Geoghegan, New York, © 1971.

Fast, J., *Body Language,* Pocket Books, New York, © 1971.

Frascone, J. and David, M., *Aphrodisiac Cook Book,* Candle Productions, Inc., Dallas, TX, © 1975.

Fulder, S., *The Tao of Medicine,* Destiny Books, New York, © 1982.

Gaynor, F., *Dictionary of Mysticism,* Citadel Press, New York, © 1968.

Gottlieb, A., *Sex Drugs and Aphrodisiacs,* Level Press, San Francisco, CA, © 1974.

Gregersen, C., *Sexual Practices, The Story of Human Sexuality,* Franklin Watts, New York, © 1983.

Haich, E., *Sexual Energy and Yoga,* ASI Publishers, Inc., New York, © 1972.

Hansen, H., *The Witch's Garden,* Unity Press, Santa Cruz, CA, © 1978.

Heffern, R., *The Complete Book of Ginseng,* Celestial Arts, Millbrae, CA, © 1976.

Hendrickson, R., *Lewd Food,* Chilton Book Co., Radnor, PA, © 1974.

Hopson, J., *Scent Signals, the Silent Language of Sex,* William Morrow and Co., New York, © 1979.

Jeanyne, *Magicks and Ceremonyes,* Lancer Books, New York, © 1972.

Liebowitz, M., *The Chemistry of Love,* Little Brown & Co., Boston, © 1983.

Lind, S. and Savary, L., *The Sleep Book,* Harper & Row, New York, © 1974.

Mann, J. (ed), *The First Book of Sacraments,* Church of The Tree of Life, San Fransisco, CA, © 1972.

Maple, E., *The Magic of Perfume,* Samuel Weiser, Inc., New York, © 1973.

Maraini, F., *Meeting with Japan,* The Viking Press, New York, © 1959.

Masters, R., *Eros and Evil: The Sexual Psychopathology of Witchcraft,* Matrix House, New York, © 1966.

Metzner, R., *Know Your Type, Maps of Identity,* Anchor Books, Garden City, NY, © 1979.

Miller, R., *The Magical and Ritual Use of Herbs,* Destiny Books, New York, © 1983.

Miller, R., *Magical Mushroom Handbook,* Homestead Press, Seattle, WA, © 1977.

Morrison, S., *The Modern Witch's Spellbook,* David McKay Co., New York, © 1971.

Mumford, J., *Sexual Occultism,* Llewellyn Publications, St. Paul, MN, © 1975.

187

Mumford, J., *Psychosomatic Yoga,* Samuel Weiser, Inc., New York, © 1974.

Ott, J., *Hallucinogenic Plants of North America,* Wingbow Press, Berkeley, CA, © 1976.

Pratt, R. and Youngken, H., *Pharmacognosy,* J.B. Lippincott Co., London, © 1951.

Riva, A., *The Modern Herbal Spellbook,* International Imports, Toluca Lake CA, © 1974.

Riviere, J., *Tantrik Yoga,* Samuel Weiser, New York, © 1970.

de Ropp, R., *Sex Energy,* Delta Books, New York, © 1969.

Schulte, R., and Hofmann, A., *The Botany and Chemistry of Hallucinogens,* Charles Thomas Publishers, Springfield, IL, © 1973.

Shalleck, J., *Tea,* The Viking Press, New York, © 1971.

Stark, R., *The Book of Aphrodisiacs,* Stein and Day, New York, © 1980.

Stone, P., *Pantheon: Archetypal Gods in Daily Living,* (unpublished), © 1984.

Stone, P., *The Holistic Qabalah: A Practical Guide to Contemporary Magick, 12 Volumes,* (unpublished), © 1984.

Superweed, M.J., *Herbal Aphrodisiacs,* Stone Kingdom Syndicate, San Francisco, CA, © 1971.

Superweed, M.J., *Herbal Highs,* Stone Kingdom Syndicate, San Francisco, CA, © 1971.

Tambimuttu, *India Love Poems,* The Peter Pauper Press, Mt. Vernon, NY, © 1967.

Twentieth Century Alchemist, *Legal Highs,* Level Press, San Francisco, CA, © 1973.

Ukers, W., *The Romance of Tea,* Alfred A. Knopf, New York, © 1936.

Veninga, L., *The Ginseng Book,* Ruka Publishing, Santa Cruz, CA, © 1973.

Walton, A., *Aphrodisiacs,* Paperback Library, New York, © 1958.

Wedeck, H., *Treasury of Witchcraft,* Philosophical Library, New York, © 1961.

Weil, A., and Winfred, R., *Chocolate to Morphine, Understanding Mind-Active Drugs,* Houghton Mifflin Co., Boston, Mass, © 1983.

Winter, R., *The Smell Book: Scents, Sex, and Society,* J.B. Lippincott Co., Philadelphia, PA, © 1976.

General Index

191

193

Chemical Index

absinthine, 102
acetal, 36
adrenalin, 126-27, 135-36
adrenergic, 116
"afrodex", 116
ajmaline, 116
alcohol, 51, 58, 62, 70, 74, 93, 103, 117, ll9, 152, 156
allergen, 12
allylpyrocathechol, 16
almond oil, 167
aloe-wood oil, 167
alpha pyrones, 58
alphoid, 68, 91
alpine rose oil, 168
aluminum, 37
ambrosia oil, 168
amino acids, 164
ammonia, 10
amphetamines, 51, 119, 150-51, 155, 157
amygdalin, 138, 162
amylase, 37
amyl nitrate, 152-53
amyris oil, 168
anabsinthin, 102
analgesic, 96, 103
androgens, 126-27, 149
antibacterial, 63
apocrine glands, 164-66
arecoline, 16, 18
artemisia oil, 168

asarone, 82-83, 86
ascorbic acid, 117, 139
atropine, 67, 90, 93

banisterine, 110
beta-asarone, 82
beta-carbolines, 108
bigonia oil, 168
biotin, 139
birch oil, 168
blood sugar, 47, 135-36
butyl nitrate, 152
B vitamins, 47, 137-39

cadinese, 16
caffeine, 44, 45
calciferol, 139
calcium, 125, 139-41
calcium oxide, 16
camellia oil, 168
camphene, 83
cannabidiolic acid, 153
cannabigerol, 153
cannabis, 153
cannibichrome, 153
carbohydrates, 135-36
cardamom oil, 168
caryophyllene, 83
cerebral cortex, 103
chavibetol, 16
chavicol, 16
chlorogenic acid, 10-12

194

chlorogenine, 10
cholinergic, 116
cholinesterase, 51
cobalt, 37
cocaine, 44, 59, 63, 119, 153-54, 156
coli bacilli, 63
copper, 37
coriander oil, 168
cortisone, 128
cyanide, 138
cyanocobalamin, 138
cyclamen oil, 168

damianian, 22
Demerol, 157
depressant, 67-68, 90-91
dextromethorphan hydrobromide, 102
dihydrokawain, 58
dihydromethysticin, 58
dihydroyangonin, 58
Dilaudid, 157
dioscin, 128
diosgenin, 128
ditaine, 10
ditamine, 10
DMSO, 154
Dolaphine, 157
dopamine, 149-50
dramamine, 52
d-tetrahydroharmine, 108

echitamine, 10
echitenines, 10
endocrine, 38
endrocrine glands, 28, 123-26
endorphins, 149
enkephalins, 149
enzyme, 51, 136, 138
epinephrine, 126
estradiol, 128
estriol, 128
estrogens, 126-28, 149
estrone, 128
ethyl mercaptan, 163
eugenol, 83
exocrine glands, 124, 126

fat solvents, 58
folacin, 139
folic acid, 139

gastric juices, 58
glutaninin acid, 37
glycosides, 36-37
gonadotrophin, 125
gonads, 126
gonococcus, 63

hallucinogen, 68, 83, 91, 116, 155
harmaline, 108-10
harmalol, 108
harmine, 108-10
hashish, 153
hawthorn oil, 168
hormones, 123-32, 138, 150
hydrobromide, 90
hyoscine, 67, 90
hyosyamine, 67, 90, 96
hypertensive crisis, 119, 155
hypnotic, 67-68, 91, 156
hypoglycemic, 135
hypotensive crisis, 119
hypothalamus gland, 125, 149-50

ibogaine, 51
indole, 51, 109, 116, 119
insulin, 126, 135-36
iproniazid, 150
iron, 37, 140
isobutyraldenhyde, 164
isopropyl alcohol, 59
isovaleric acid, 164

kawaine, 58, 63

lactucarine, 96
lactucerol, 96
lactucic acid, 96
lactucin, 96
laetrile, 138
laudanum oil, 168
L-Dopa, 128, 155
lecithin, 59, 140
levodopa, 155
LHRH, 126, 150

195

196

Also by Richard Alan Miller,

the companion volume to
The Magical & Ritual Use of Aphrodisiacs:

THE MAGICAL & RITUAL
USE OF HERBS

This highly sophisticated study of nineteen stimulant, depressant, narcotic, and hallucinogenic herbs is written by
an expert for those who are seeking authoritative information on the practical and magical uses of these substances.
It provides a wealth of historical background, chemical
descriptions and diagrams, and instructions for the preparation, consumption, and ritual application of each of the
herbs.

The author explains how to use specific herbs to stimulate sexual energies, combat fatigue, assist the healing
process, relieve tension, and promote feelings of well-being
and self-awareness. Details are also given on herbal preparations that are ideally suited to relaxation and massage,
initiation and spiritual growth, and the performing of
sacraments for astral projection.

ISBN: 0-89281-047-5   *Quality Paperback*   *$6.95*